SV-40 VIRUSES

Papers by
Keerti V. Shah, Hilary Koprowski, Hiroshi Yamamoto, Ronald Duff, Richard W. Smith, Miriam Margalith, Wanda Baranska, Richard G. Olsen, Mary C. Weiss, C.W. Potter, Satvir S. Tevethia, Chou-Chik Ting, John R. Sheppard, Michael P. Friedman, M. Nachtigal, Hannah Ben-Bassat, David M. Trilling, Klaus Hummeler, Giuseppe Barbanti-Brodano et al.

MSS Information Corporation
655 Madison Avenue, New York, N.Y. 10021

Library of Congress Cataloging in Publication Data

Main entry under title:

SV-40 viruses.

    1. Simian vacuolating virus--Addresses, essays,
lectures. I. Shah   Keerti V. [DNLM: 1. SV40
virus--Collected works. QW 160.S8 S112 1973]
QR360.S18   576'.6484   72-13566
ISBN 0-8422-7064-7

TABLE OF CONTENTS

CREDITS AND ACKNOWLEDGEMENTS

Baranska, Wanda; Pavel Koldovsky; and Hilary Koprowski, "Antigenic Study of Unfertilized Mouse Eggs: Cross Reactivity with SV40-Induced Antigens," *Proceedings of the National Academy of Sciences*, 1970, 67:193-199.

Barbanti-Brodano, Giuseppe; Peter Swetly; and Hilary Koprowski, "Early Events in the Infection of Permissive Cells with Simian Virus 40: Adsorption, Penetration, and Uncoating," *Journal of Virology*, 1970, 6:78-86.

Ben-Bassat, Hannah; Michael Inbar; and Leo Sachs, "Requirement for Cell Replication after SV40 Infection for a Structural Change of the Cell Surface Membrane," *Virology*, 1970, 40:854-859.

Duff, Ronald; and Fred Rapp, "Reaction of Serum from Pregnant Hamsters with Surface Cells Transformed by SV40," *The Journal of Immunology*, 1970, 105:521-523.

Duff, Ronald; Fred Rapp; and Janet S. Butel, "Transformation of Hamster Cells by Variants of PARA-Adenovirus 7 Able to Induce SV40 Tumor Antigen in the Cytoplasm," *Virology*, 1970, 42:273-275.

Friedman, Michael P.; Michael J. Lyons; and Harold S. Ginsberg, Biochemical Consequences of Type 2 Adenovirus and Simian Virus 40 Double Infections of African Green Monkey Kidney Cells," *Journal of Virology*, 1970, 5:586-597.

Hummeler, Klaus; Natale Tomassini; and Frantisek Sokol, "Morphological Aspects of the Uptake of Simian Virus 40 by Permissive Cells," *Journal of Virology*, 1970, 6:87-93.

Koprowski, Hilary; Wojciech Sawicki; and Pavel Koldovsky, "Immunologic Cross-Reactivity Between Antigen of Unfertilized Mouse Eggs and Mouse Cells Transformed by Simian Virus 40," *Journal of the National Cancer Institute*, 1971, 46:1317-1323.

Margalith, Miriam; Eva Margalith; Tamar Nasialski; and N. Goldblum, "Induction of Simian Virus 40 Antigen in BSC$_1$ Transformed Cells," *Journal of Virology*, 1970, 5:305-308.

Nachtigal, Maurice; Joseph L. Melnick; and Janet S. Butel, "Chromosomal Changes in Syrian Hamster Cells Transformed by Simian Virus 40 (SV40) and Variants of Defective SV40 (PARA)," *Journal of the National Cancer Institute*, 1971, 47:35-45.

Nachtigal, M.; and J.S. Butel, "Variation in Response of Syrian Hamster Lung Cells to Complete or Defective SV40 (PARA)," *Proceedings of the Society for Experimental Biology and Medicine*, 1970, 135:727-731.

Olsen, Richard G.; James R. McCammon; Joseph Weber; and David S. Yohn, "Cutaneous Skin Test for Delayed Hypersensitivity in Hamsters to Viral Induced Tumor Antigens," *Canadian Journal of Microbiology*, 1971, 17:1145-1147.

Potter, C.W.; A.M. Potter; and J.S. Oxford, "Comparison of Transformation and T Antigen Induction in Human Cell Lines," *Journal of Virology*, 1970, 5:293-298.

Shah, Keerti V.; Harvey L. Ozer; Harry S. Pond; Loreto D. Palma; and Gerald P. Murphy, "SV40 Neutralizing Antibodies in Sera of U.S. Residents Without History of Polio Immunization," *Nature*, 1971, 231:448-449.

Shah, Keerti V.; Manohar K. Goverdhan; and Harvey L. Ozer, "Neutralizing Antibodies to SV40 in Human Sera from South India: Search for Additional Hosts of SV40," *American Journal of Epidemiology*, 1971, 93:291-297.

Sheppard, John R.; Arnold J. Levine; and Max M. Burger, "Cell-Surface Changes after Infection with Oncogenic Viruses: Requirement for Synthesis of Host DNA," *Science*, 1971, 172:1345-1346.

Smith, Richard W.; Joel Morganroth; and Peter T. Mora, "SV40 Virus-Induced Tumour Specific Transplantation Antigen in Cultured Mouse Cells," *Nature*, 1970, 227:141-145.

Tevethia, Satvir S.; Norman A. Crouch; Joseph L. Melnick; and Fred Rapp, "Detection of Specific Surface Antigens by Colony Inhibition in Cells Transformed by Papovavirus SV40," *International Journal of Cancer*, 1970, 5:176-184.

Ting, Chou-Chik; and Ronald B. Herberman, "Detection of Tumor-Specific Cell Surface Antigen of Simian Virus 40-Induced Tumors by the Isotopic Antiglobulin Technique," *International Journal of Cancer*, 1971, 7:499-506.

Trilling, David M.; and David Axelrod, "Encapsidation of Free Host DNA by Simian Virus 40: A Simian Virus 40 Pseudovirus," *Science*, 1970, 168:268-271.

Weiss, Mary C., "Further Studies on Loss of T-Antigen from Somatic Hybrids Between Mouse Cells and SV40-Transformed Human Cells," *Proceedings of the National Academy of Sciences*, 1970, 66:79-86.

Yamamoto, Hiroshi; and Hiroto Shimojo, "Inactivation of T Antigen-Forming Capacities of Simian Virus 40 and Adenovirus 12 by Ultraviolet Irradiation," *Journal of Virology*, 1971, 7:419-425.

PREFACE

SV-40 (simian Papovavirus), a subject of intense research to-day, represents one of the most accessible model systems for the study of virus-mediated oncogenic transformation.

Studies on the effects of SV-40 viruses on tissue culture cells are underway at various levels including experimentation with viral nucleic acid metabolism, and viral effects on host cell behavior and host cell components. Nucleic acid and protein components of the virion, as well as the nature of integration of the viral genome into the host cell, are also being analyzed.

The present three-volume collection includes articles, published from 1970-1972, dealing with these and related topics.

Antigenic Relationships of SV-40

SV40 Neutralizing Antibodies in Sera of US Residents without History of Polio Immunization

Keerti V. Shah
Harvey L. Ozer
Harry S. Pond
Loreto D. Palma
Gerald P. Murphy

Simian virus 40 (SV40) is a natural infection of rhesus and some other Asiatic macaques[1] and has no known natural host in the United States. It is therefore difficult to account for our finding of antibodies neutralizing SV40 in the sera of some elderly persons in the United States who do not have a history of immunization with any vaccine prepared in rhesus kidney cultures. The only recognized exposure of the US population to this virus occurred when poliovirus and adenovirus vaccines prepared in rhesus kidney cultures and administered to a large number of people were later found to have been contaminated with SV40 (ref. 1). The chief exposure occurred between 1955 and 1961 through the use of Salk vaccine, and it is known that subcutaneous administration of SV40 gives a long-lasting antibody response[2].

We made our observations during a continuing study of cancer of the urinary bladder in a search for possible papovavirus aetiology. Sera from 210 patients with bladder or other types of cancer were screened for antibodies to SV40. The donors comprised 157 white males, thirty-seven white females, fifteen negro males and one negro female and had a median age of 66.

The sera were initially screened at 1 : 2 dilution in SV40 virus neutralization tests[3]. Antibodies were detected in sera of two of eight Salk vaccinees and in seven of 184 who gave a history of no immunization. These latter seven donors, six white males and one white female, were interviewed in detail about their immunization history and were bled periodically

This work was supported by grants from the American Cancer Society, the National Institutes of Health and the National Chapter of Phi Beta Phi Sorority.

10

Table 1 Presence of SV40 Antibodies in Sera of Cancer Patients

Patient	Age	Sex	Date of bleeding	Neutral. antibody titre	FA-viral antibody titre	RIP value (% virus precipitated) serum dilution 1:20	1:100	Diagnosis and status of disease
N. H.	68	M	6-21-69	1:8	1:2	27	16	Carcinoma prostate, treated June and August 1969
			9-17-69	1:8	1:4	33	14	
			4-13-70	1:2	1:1	24	—	
C. D.	56	M	6-10-69	1:8	1:32	46	16	Treated carcinoma bladder. No recurrence, 1 yr
			9-9-69	1:8	1:32	49	17	
			5-26-70	1:4	1:16	55	—	
L. G.	66	M	5-24-69	1:8	Negative	—	5	Treated carcinoma bladder. No recurrence, 4 yr
			9-17-69	1:4	Negative	5	3	
H. G.	69	M	6-26-69	1:16	1:1	29	13	Treated carcinoma bladder. No recurrence, 5 yr
			8-24-69	1:32	1:1	26	14	
			3-10-70	1:32	1:1	18	—	
W. C.	50	M	6-22-69	1:4	Negative	6	6	Treated seminoma testes. No recurrence, 3 yr
			5-26-70	1:4	Negative	7	—	
C. C.	58	F	9-12-69	1:64	1:8	62	25	Follicular lymphosarcoma. Treated October 1969
			2-18-70	1:64	1:2	24	—	
G. H.	74	M	1-29-70	1:32	Negative	10	—	Carcinoma prostate, persistent, 3 yr
			6-5-70	1:32	Negative	19	—	

Antibodies to SV40 in repeated bleedings of seven individuals without history of poliovirus immunization. Results of only some of the collected sera are given. A serum was interpreted as staining SV40 viral antigen in fluorescent antibody tests if (a) there was nuclear fluorescence of at least 1 + intensity in the appropriate proportion of cells; (b) the serum did not stain uninfected cells; and (c) the staining was inhibited by previous treatment of the cultures with FUDR. For determination of T antibodies, sera were reacted against SV40-transformed hamster cells and against FUDR-treated acutely infected cells. An RIP value (% virus precipitated) of 12% was considered positive. Eleven neutralization negative sera had RIP values of 0–6%. A hyperimmune monkey anti-SV40 serum gave 60–80% precipitation.

for antibody determination in neutralization, fluorescent antibody[4] and radioisotope precipitation (RIP) tests[5].

All seven affirmed that they had not received any kind of poliovaccine. Detailed questioning provided no evidence that any of them was either immunized with an experimental vaccine or was exposed to a known source of SV40 in his occupation or travel. Antibody levels in different bleedings of the same individual were comparable (Table 1). Neutralizing antibody titres in different individuals ranged from 1 : 2 to 1 : 64. Sera from four persons specifically and consistently stained SV40 viral antigen in indirect fluorescent antibody tests. With the exception of sera from C. D., which had titres of 1 : 16 and 1 : 32, antibody titres in fluorescent antibody tests were low. None of the approximately 200 neutralization negative sera stained the viral antigen, thus indicating the specificity of the reaction. None of the sera, including those from C. D., stained SV40 T antigen. The results of RIP tests generally supported the neutralization and fluorescent antibody studies. The sera of N. H., C. D., H. G., and C. C., at 1 : 20 dilution consistently gave precipitation values well above the 12% used in the past to define a positive serum[6]. These sera were also positive in both neutralization and fluorescent antibody tests. In all cases tested, sera which were positive at 1 : 20 dilution were also positive at 1 : 100 dilution, though with lower values (Table 1).

The evidence for the presence of SV40-reacting antibodies in most of the individuals listed in Table 1 is unequivocal. These included patients with different malignant diseases, active or inactive. Other preliminary studies do not suggest a higher prevalence of antibodies in patients with cancer of the bladder than in any other diagnostic category[7]. Although it is impossible to exclude the possibility that the donors, in spite of their history, were immunized with Salk vaccine, several considerations make this unlikely. It has been estimated that only about 10% of the non-institutionalized civilian population aged 50–59 yr had received one or more inoculations of Salk vaccine by September 1961 (ref. 8); the median age of our subjects was 58 yr in 1961. Furthermore, not all lots of Salk vaccine were contaminated with SV40 (ref. 9) and not all people who received contaminated vaccine uniformly developed SV40 antibodies[1,2].

In earlier investigations[3,4], one of us reported the detection of SV40 neutralizing antibodies in sera of normal and cancerous individuals in North India not immunized with poliovaccine and had interpreted this to indicate natural transmission of SV40 from the resident rhesus population to man. Although this interpretation may still be correct, our findings, as well as the recent detection of SV40 antibodies in human sera from South India where rhesus is not prevalent[6], raise the possibility of alternative explanations. The antibodies may be the result of infection with a related papovavirus. Papovaviruses known to infect man include the wart virus and the virus seen by electron microscopy in lesions of progressive multifocal leucoencephalopathy[10]. There are also reports of isolation of

12

papova-like viruses from human brains of Creutzfeld-Jacob disease[11] and subacute sclerosing panencephalitis[12]. It is not known whether infection with any of these agents will produce antibodies which will react with SV40 virion. There may be natural hosts of SV40 other than Asiatic macaques or the antibodies may be a result of infection with a hitherto undescribed SV40-like infection of man.

[1] Sweet, B. H., and Hilleman, M. R., *Proc. Soc. Exp. Biol. Med.*, **105**, 420 (1960).
[2] Gerber, P., *Proc. Soc. Exp. Biol. Med.*, **125**, 1284 (1967).
[3] Shah, K. V., *Proc. Soc. Exp. Biol. Med.*, **121**, 303 (1966).
[4] Shah, K. V., *J. Nat. Cancer Inst.*, **14**, 139 (1969).
[5] Ozer, H. L., Takemoto, K. K., Kirschstein, R. L., and Axelrod, D., *Virology*, **3** (1), 17 (1969).
[6] Shah, K. V., Goverdhan, M. K., and Ozer, H. L., *Amer. J. Epidemiol.*, **93**, 291 (1971).
[7] Shah, K. V., Palma, L. D., and Murphy, G. P., *J. Surg. Oncol.*, **3** (in the press).
[8] *CDC, USPHS, Polio Surveillance Reports*, Report No. 248, 5 (1961).
[9] Gerber, P., Hottle, G. A., and Grubbs, R. E., *Proc. Soc. Exp. Biol. Med.*, **108**, 205 (1961).
[10] Zu Rhein, G., *Prog. Med. Virol.*, **11**, 185 (1969).
[11] Vernon, M. L., Fuccillo, D. A., and Hamilton, R., *Fed. Proc.*, **29**, No. 229 (1970).
[12] Koprowski, H., Barbanti-Brodano, G., and Katz, M., *Nature*, **225**, 1045 (1970).

NEUTRALIZING ANTIBODIES TO SV40 IN HUMAN SERA FROM SOUTH INDIA: SEARCH FOR ADDITIONAL HOSTS OF SV40

KEERTI V. SHAH, MANOHAR K. GOVERDHAN AND HARVEY L. OZER[1]

In earlier investigations (1, 2), one of us described the finding of neutralizing antibodies to SV40 in a proportion of human sera from North India. Antibodies were present in low titers and were detected in 8.7 per cent of noncancerous residents of Uttar Pradesh (1) and in 5.3 per cent of cancer patients in North India (2). In addi-

[1] From the Department of Pathobiology, School of Hygiene and Public Health, The Johns Hopkins University, Baltimore, Maryland (Dr. Shah); Virus Research Center, Poona, India (Dr. Goverdhan); and Laboratory of Biochemistry, National Cancer Institute, National Institutes of Health, Bethesda, Maryland 20014 (Dr. Ozer). The authors gratefully acknowledge the help of Dr. S. Krishnamurthi, and Dr. S. Sankaran of the Cancer Institute, Madras; Dr. H. S. Bhat, Dr. Padam Singh, and Dr. P. Venugopal of the Christian Medical College and Hospital, Vellore, in collection of the human sera; Dr. T. R. Rao, Director, Virus Research Center, Poona, in providing the animal sera; and Dr. Fred Hymes, Immunoglobulin Reference Center, in providing the antiglobulin for RIP tests. Supported by Grant E440A from the American Cancer Society and by USPHS Grant 5 RO7 TW00141-09 CIC from NIH to The Johns Hopkins Center for Medical Research and Training.

tion, 27 per cent of individuals who cared for large numbers of juvenile rhesus for monkey export firms had SV40 neutralizing antibodies (1).

All of the above individuals lived inside the known limits of the distribution of the rhesus monkey (*Macaca mulatta*), the natural host of SV40, and none gave history of immunization with any vaccine prepared in monkey kidney. Since there are no known cross-reactions between SV40 and other viruses in neutralization tests, the above findings were interpreted as indicating natural infection of man with SV40.

In this communication, we report the detection of SV40 neutralizing antibodies in a proportion of sera of cancer patients from South India who live several hundred miles away from the southern limits of rhesus distribution. Sera from six animal species of South India—including bonnet and langur monkeys, the two most prevalent monkeys in this region—were also screened for SV40 neutralizing antibodies. Human sera from both North and South India were further evaluated by the radioisotope immunoprecipitation (RIP) test with SV40.

MATERIALS AND METHODS

Sera from South Indian cancer patients. A total of 155 sera were collected from two hospitals in South India, the Cancer Institute, Madras, and the Christian Medical College and Hospital, Vellore. Both of these hospitals are located in the state of Tamil Nadu, and are situated more than 300 miles south of the lower limit of rhesus distribution (figure 1). Notes were made of the age, sex, duration of illness, diagnosis and state of residence of the patient. It was ascertained that most of the patients had never visited North India. None gave history of vaccination against poliomyelitis.

Animal sera. A total of 250 sera from Mysore State, South India, collected by the staff of the Virus Research Center, Poona, India, were tested for neutralizing antibodies to SV40. Sera were initially screened at the dilution of 1:3. They were from six species: 50 each from the bonnet (*Macaca radiata*) and langur (*Presbytis entellus*) monkeys, 25 each from cow and buffalo, and 50 each from goat and sheep. The age of the donor animals is indicated with the results of the tests.

Neutralization tests. Neutralization tests were performed as previously described (1) in roller tubes of primary African Green

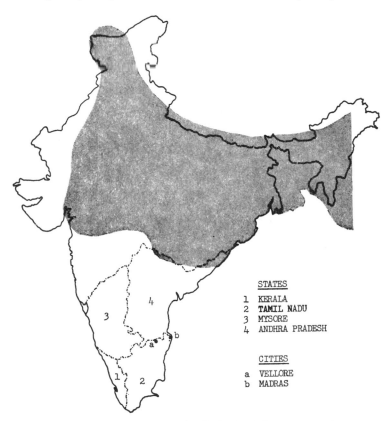

STATES

1 KERALA
2 **TAMIL NADU**
3 MYSORE
4 ANDHRA PRADESH

CITIES

a VELLORE
b MADRAS

Figure 1. Map of India showing rhesus distribution (shaded area) and localities of serum collection.

15

TABLE 1

Prevalence of SV40 neutralizing antibodies by age and sex of donor

Age in years	Males		Females	
	No. tested	No. with antibodies	No. tested	No. with antibodies
20–29	6	1	5	0
30–39	10	2	11	0
40–49	18	2	26	3
50–59	22	1	30	0
60–69	10	0	12	0
70+	2	1	—	—
Total	68	7 (10.3%)	84	3 (3.6%)

Total No. with antibodies 10 (6.5%)

Total males and females 155*

* Three individuals of unrecorded age, all without antibodies, included.

monkey kidney (AGMK) cells. Sera inactivated at 56 C for 30 minutes were initially tested undiluted or at 1:2 dilution and those showing neutralization were titrated with twofold dilutions. Serum-virus mixtures were incubated at 37 C for 45 minutes and then overnight at 4 C. Interpretations were made when the effective virus dose was at least 30 TCD_{50}.

Fluorescent antibody (FA) tests. All human sera and some of the animal sera were tested in indirect FA tests with AGMK cells acutely infected with SV40 for the presence of SV40 viral and T antibodies. The preparation of the antigens and other reagents and the details of the test have been described before (2).

Radioisotope immunoprecipitation test (RIP). The RIP test, which measures the ability of sera to precipitate radiolabeled purified virus in the presence of antiglobulin, was performed as described by Ozer et al. (3). Selected sera from North and South India were diluted 1:10 in phosphate buffered saline (PBS), coded and stored frozen. Prior to testing, all sera were centrifuged at 10,000 × g for five minutes to remove aggregates and diluted to a final concentration of 1:100 in 0.1 per cent BSA, 0.15 M NaCl, 0.02

M Tris, pH 7.4. Antiglobulin (goat anti-human IgG) was used at a 1:5 dilution.

SV40 was radioactively labeled with thymidine or amino acids as previously described (3). Both preparations (500 counts per minute cpm per test) showed 50 per cent precipitation with a monkey anti-SV40 serum diluted 1:100. It should be noted that at the antiglobulin:anti-SV40 serum ratio used, less than maximal precipitation was observed. Samples were counted in Triton-Toluene by liquid scintillation spectroscopy (4). A serum was considered positive if an average of at least two determinations of precipitation was greater than 12 per cent.

RIP inhibition was performed as previously described using 20 micrograms of purified unlabelled SV40.

RESULTS

Neutralizing antibodies in human sera. Ten of 155 sera (6.5 per cent) from South Indian cancer patients had neutralizing antibodies to SV40 (table 1). All patients were adults and the protective sera were scattered in the different age groups. There was a somewhat higher prevalence in males. All donors of protective sera were residents of one or another of the South Indian states (table 2) which are outside the limits of rhesus distribution (figure 1).

TABLE 2

Prevalence of SV40 neutralizing antibodies by donor's residence

State of residence*	No. tested	No. with antibodies
Tamil Nadu	92	5
Andhra Pradesh	38	0
Kerala	12	4
Mysore	3	1
Assam	4	0
Orissa	1	0
Total	150	10

* One individual from Nepal and four individuals with state of residence not recorded, were excluded; all these were without antibodies.

16

TABLE 3

Prevalence of SV40 neutralizing antibodies in sera of patients by site or type of tumor

Site or type of tumor	No. of sera tested	No. of sera with anti-bodies	Antibody titers of positive sera
Oral cavity	60	3	1:2, 1:4, 1:4
Pharynx	6	1	1:4
Gastrointestinal tract	10	0	—
Lymphatic system	4	0	—
Respiratory tract	7	2	1:8, 1:32
Cancer cervix	43	2	1:2, 1:4
Cancer urinary bladder	8	2	1:8, 1:8
External genitals	5	0	—
Others	12	0	—
	155	10	

The prevalence of neutralizing antibodies by site or type of tumor and titers of the protective sera are given in table 3. There was no preponderance of protective sera in any of the diagnostic categories. Antibody titers were low and only four of 10 sera had titers of 1:8 or greater.

Fluorescent antibody (FA) tests of human sera. In indirect FA tests against AGMK cells acutely infected with SV40, none of the sera were shown to have SV40 viral or T antibodies. The protective sera were also negative for T antibodies in tests with SV40-transformed hamster cells which have T antigen in nuclei of 100 per cent of the cells.

Evaluation of the neutralizing activity of sera from North and South India. The low titers of neutralizing antibodies in protective sera and the finding of such sera in South India where rhesus is not prevalent required a careful evaluation of the specificity of the neutralizing activity in Indian sera. The following is a summary of these efforts.

Reproducibility. The sera were always inactivated at 56 C for 30 minutes for neutralization tests. All sera listed as protective were tested at least twice and some tive were tested at least twice and some as many as six times. Tests were read blind. Results of tests both of protective and negative sera were reproducible. Plaque reduction neutralization tests (5) were performed on 40 sera, 10 of them protective by neutralization tests. There was complete correspondence between the results of the two tests in terms of protective and negative sera; plaque reduction neutralization titers were higher.

Specificity. Sera protective against SV40 did not neutralize polyoma virus. None of 19 sera, nine of them protective against SV40, neutralized 50 $TCID_{50}$ of polyoma virus in tests in mouse embryo tissue culture. In tests in AGMK cultures, SV40-protective sera did not neutralize simian adenoviruses SA7 and SV20 more often than negative sera.

Attempts to increase sensitivity. Two techniques were tried in an attempt to increase the efficiency of neutralization. In the first, the virus to be used in neutralization tests was passed through a 100 mμ gradocol filter to remove aggregates. Such filtration has been shown to increase the efficiency of neutralization of an enterovirus (6). In the second, an antiglobulin neutralization test (AGN) was performed. AGN tests have been shown to increase the sensitivity of neutralizing activity against herpes simplex and arboviruses (7, 8). The initial period of incubation of serum-virus mixture was followed by addition of anti-human gamma globulin and further incubation for one hour at 37 C; 0.2 ml of a 1:5 dilution of rabbit anti-human IgG (Melpar Laboratories) was added to 0.4 ml of serum-virus mixture. Neither the prior filtration of test virus nor the addition of antiglobulin to serum-virus mixture increased the efficiency of virus neutralization by 10 protective sera.

RIP tests. The comparison of results of RIP and neutralization tests is given in table 4. As described in Material and Methods, sera were diluted 1:100 and the test measured only IgG antibodies. Significant precipitation of radioactive virus occurred with four neutralization-positive sera. These sera, all of them from North India, were among the nine with neutralizing antibody titers of 1:16 or 1:32. Of the four sera which were both FA and neutralization test positive, two were RIP positive. The highest RIP value obtained for a human serum was 51 per cent (25 per cent at a dilution of 1:500), a value as high as that of the immune monkey serum. The donor was a 50-year-old male from North India with cancer of the penis.

The three human sera with RIP values of 17, 25, and 51 per cent were further evaluated to rule out nonspecific precipitation. None of them precipitated virus in the absence of antiglobulin and, in all cases, precipitation of the labeled virus was inhibited by addition of an excess of unlabeled purified SV40.

The RIP values of the 20 neutralization test negative as well as of the 10 sera with antibody titers between 1:2 and 1:8 ranged from 0 to 10 per cent. When retested at a 1:20 dilution of serum (using undiluted antiglobulin) these sera give a RIP value of 0, thus supporting the conclusion that an isolated RIP value of 10 per cent was not significant under the conditions of the test.

Neutralization tests of animal sera from South India. Since the rhesus range does not extend to South India, the presence of neutralizing antibodies in human sera from South India suggested some other host of SV40 in this area. Two hundred and fifty animal sera from South India were screened for neutralizing antibodies to SV40. These included 50 sera from each of the two common monkeys in South India, the South Indian bonnet macaque, *Macaca radiata* and the langur, *Presbytis entellus*.

The results are given in table 5. The 100 sera from the two monkey species were all clearly negative as also the 25 sera from buffalo. The results with cow, sheep and goat sera were difficult to interpret as a number of them variably delayed the onset or the progression of SV40 cytopathic effect by one to three days and could not be

TABLE 4

Comparison of RIP and neutralization test results

	No. of sera with neutralizing antibody titers						
	Neg.	1:1	1:2	1:4	1:8	1:16	1:32
North India	2	0	1	2	0	3	5
South India	18	0	1	4	2	0	1
Total	20	0	2	6	2	3	6
Positive in RIP	0	0	0	0	0	2	2
Average % precipitation of each positive serum						13, 17	25, 51

clearly classified as protective or negative. The inhibitory effect was not present at dilutions above 1:8. Sixteen of these sera (eight of 25 cow sera, five of 50 goat sera and three of 50 sheep sera) which showed the maximum inhibitory effect were tested in indirect FA tests with AGMK cells acutely infected with SV40; none stained viral or T antigen.

DISCUSSION

In many respects, the pattern of occurrence of SV40 neutralizing antibodies in sera of cancer patients from South India resembled that described earlier for cancerous and noncancerous residents of North India. The antibody prevalence of 6.5 per cent in South Indian patients was similar to the 5.3 prevalence in North Indian cancerous patients (2) and to the 8.7 per cent

TABLE 5

Results of tests for neutralizing antibodies to SV40 in sera of monkeys and other animals from Mysore State, South India

Species*	Age	No. tested	No. with anti-bodies
Bonnet (*Macaca radiata*)	Juvenile	50	0
Langur (*Presbytis antellus*)	Adult	50	0
Buffalo	3–12 years	25	0

* Low level inhibition of SV40 cytopathic effect shown by eight of 25 cow sera, five of 50 goat sera and three of 50 sheep sera. Specificity of this reaction is under investigation.

prevalence in North Indian noncancerous individuals (1). Further, the protective sera in all three groups had low titers of neutralizing antibodies, no T antibodies, and were scattered in the different age groups.

It is very unlikely that rhesus is the source of SV40 infection of this South Indian population. The southern limit of the known distribution of rhesus is several hundred miles north of the localities where the sera were collected and most of the serum donors, including those with neutralizing antibodies, did not give a history of visiting North India. A few rhesus, probably introduced, have been sighted in South India outside the range shown in figure 1, but they are too few to be of any significance as a source of SV40 infection.

In consideration of natural animal hosts of SV40 in South India, the two most common monkeys in the South, the bonnet macaque and the black-faced langur, appeared to be the most likely possibilities. Asiatic macaques are the only known natural hosts of SV40: *M. mulatta* in India and in North Viet Nam (9, 10), *M. fuscata* in Japan (11), *M. cylopis* in Taiwan (12), and the cynomolgous monkey, *M. fascicularis* (13, 14) in East Asia. The bonnet, *Macaca radiata*, is a close relative of rhesus, occupies the same ecological niche in South India as the rhesus does in the north, often lives close to human communities and is probably the most abundant of the South Indian monkeys. The langur, *Presbytis entellus*, is found throughout India and its distribution overlaps with that of rhesus in North India.

However, there was no evidence of natural infection of either the bonnet or the langur with SV40. We did not detect neutralizing antibodies in 50 sera from each of these species, mostly from adults, collected from animals in Mysore State. Sera from bonnet in two other localities in South India have been tested previously in other laboratories. At the Pasteur Institute, Coonoor, where bonnet kidneys are routinely used for the production of poliovaccine, Bala-

subramanian et al. (15) have not found SV40 neutralizing antibodies in tests of 143 bonnet sera or encountered SV40 virus in bonnet kidney cultures. Similarly, John et al. (16) found 83 sera from juvenile bonnet, collected from around Vellore, Tamil Nadu State, negative for SV40 neutralizing antibodies.

Apart from the bonnet, the only other macaque in South India is *Macaca sileneus*, the lion-tailed macaque. This species is rare and its distribution is limited to a few areas in high altitude forests (17).

One of the major problems in the interpretation of results with human sera was the low titers of protective sera. Attempts to increase the sensitivity of the neutralization test were not successful. We have tended to accept the low titers as due to viral antibody for two reasons: (a) nonantibody inhibitors of SV40 have not been described in human sera, and (b) except when given by the subcutaneous route (18), SV40 elicits only a low-grade or minimal antibody response in man (19, 20).

In reports of earlier investigations, we have described the finding of SV40 neutralizing antibodies in human sera from North India (1, 2) and confirmation of the neutralization test results of some of these sera by FA tests (2). Analysis of the sera for antibodies to SV40 virion by precipitation of radioactively labeled purified virus (RIP) confirmed the presence of viral antibodies in four North Indian sera. These were among the nine sera, eight of them from North India, which had neutralizing antibody titers of 1:16 or 1:32. The inability to test sera in the RIP at dilutions less than 1:20 would be expected to preclude the confirmation of many of the low titered neutralizing positive sera.

It should be pointed out that the results of FA and RIP tests confirmed none of the neutralization-positive sera from South India. This may be because there were only 10 such sera in the South Indian sample, all but one with titers of 1:8 or less. In view of these data, and the lack of an identifiable reservoir of SV40 in the South, we suggest caution in the interpretation of neutralization test results of South Indian sera.

The possibility that the low-level neutralization of SV40 is a result of infection with an antigenically related papovavirus should be considered. The only well characterized papovavirus of man is the wart virus. Melnick and Rapp (21) have reported that hamsters immunized with wart virus resisted challenge with SV40-transformed cells. We have not been able to test the SV40 protective Indian sera for wart antibodies. Another papovavirus which appears to be clearly associated with man is the virus detected by electron microscopy in the affected sites of brain in progressive multifocal leucoencephalopathy (PML) (22). It is not known if this virus has any antigenic relationship with SV40.

In the study of North Indian cancer patients (2), a somewhat higher prevalence of SV40 neutralizing antibodies was found in patients with cancer of the urinary bladder. In the present investigation, two of eight patients with bladder cancer in South India had SV40 neutralizing antibodies. A detailed investigation of cancer of the urinary bladder for possible papovavirus etiology will be described separately.

REFERENCES

1. Shah KV: Neutralizing antibodies to simian virus 40 (SV40) in human sera from India. Proc Soc Exp Biol Med 121: 303–307, 1966
2. Shah KV: Investigation of human malignant tumors in India for SV40 etiology. J Nat Cancer Inst 42: 139–145, 1969
3. John TJ, Feldman RA, Tsuchiya Y: Personal communication, 1968
4. Patterson MS, Greene RC: Measurement of low energy beta-emitters in aqueous solution by liquid scintillation counting of emulsions. Anal Chem 37: 854–857, 1965
5. Stinebaugh S, Melnick JL: Plaque formation by vacuolating virus, SV40. Virology 16: 348–349, 1962
6. Wallis C, Melnick JL: Virus aggregation as the cause of the non-neutralizable persistent fraction. J Virol 1: 478–488, 1967
7. Notkins AL, Makar S, Scheele C, et al: Infectious virus-antibody complex in the blood of chronically infected mice. J Exp Med 124: 81–97, 1966
8. Brown A, Elsner V, Zebovits E, et al: Use of an antiglobulin plaque neutralization test among group A arboviruses. Proc Soc Exp Biol Med 130: 718–722, 1969
9. Shah KV, Southwick CH: Prevalence of antibodies to certain viruses in sera of free-living rhesus and of captive monkeys. Indian J Med Res 53: 488–500, 1965
10. Lapin BA, Dzhikidze EK, Yakovlova LA, et al: Infection of monkeys with SV40 virus in the jungles of North Vietnam. Vop Virus 2: 226–228, 1965
11. Personal communication from Dr. Y. Tsuchiya, 1965
12. Yang CS, Kuo CH, Chen CY: A study on natural infection of simian virus 40 (SV40) in Taiwan monkeys (*Macaca cyclopis*). J Formosan Med Assoc 66: 43–48, 1967
13. Meyer HM Jr, Hopps HE, Rogers NG, et al: Studies on simian virus 40. J Immunol 88: 796–806, 1962
14. Tsuchiya Y: Personal communication, 1969
15. Balasubramanian A, Vijayan P, Lingan H, et al: Annual Report of the Director, 1966, and Scientific Report, 1967. The Pasteur Institute of Southern India, Coonoor.
16. John TJ, Feldman RA, Tsuchiya Y: Personal communication, 1968
17. Sugiyama Y: The ecology of the lion-tailed macaque (*Macaca sileneus*, Linnaeus): a pilot study. J Bombay Nat Hist Soc 65: 283, 1968
18. Sweet BH, Hilleman MR: The vacuolating virus, SV40. Proc Soc Exp Biol Med 105: 420–427, 1960
19. Morris JA, Johnson KM, Aulisio CG, et al: Clinical and serologic responses in volunteer given vacuolating virus (SV40) by respiratory route. Proc Soc Exp Biol Med 108: 56–59, 1961
20. Melnick JL, Stinebaugh S: Excretion of vacuolating SV40 virus (papova virus group) after ingestion as a contaminant of oral poliovaccine. Proc Soc Exp Biol Med 109: 965–968, 1962
21. Melnick JL, Rapp F: Possible relationship between two primate papovaviruses, human wart and simian virus 40. J Nat Cancer Inst 34: 529–534, 1965
22. Zu Rhein G: Association of papova-virions with a human demyelinating disease (progressive multifocal leucoencephalopathy). Progr Med Virol 11: 185–247, 1969

Immunologic Cross-Reactivity Between Antigen of Unfertilized Mouse Eggs and Mouse Cells Transformed by Simian Virus 40[1]

Hilary Koprowski, Wojciech Sawicki, *and* Pavel Koldovsky,

IN PRELIMINARY studies (*1*), we reported that antibody obtained from guinea pigs immunized with unfertilized one celled mouse eggs was cytotoxic for mouse cells transformed by simian virus 40 (SV40), but not for cells of adult mice.

This embryonic antigen in cells transformed by the oncogenic SV40 falls into a category of carcinoembryonic antigens that can be detected either by transplantation reaction or by direct cytotoxicity test (*e.g.*, *2*). In this ill-defined group, older embryos, rather than unfertilized one-celled eggs, were used as a source of antigen for cross-reactivity purposes. Thus it is difficult to compare directly the results obtained with SV40-egg antigen to those obtained with other tumor-embryo combinations. We know, however, that we are dealing with cell surface antigens differing considerably from the other two categories of cancer-embryonic antigens. One category includes the α-globulin secreted by hepatoma cells and found also in sera of mice at birth in quantities that decrease gradually during postnatal life (*3*). The other category includes the antigen described by Gold and Freedman (*4*) in human malignant tumors of endo-

[1] Supported in part by Public Health Service research grants P01-CA 10815 and R01-CA 04534 from the National Cancer Institute, S01-RR 05540 from the General Research Support Branch, and funds from the Lalor Foundation.

dermis-derived epithelium of the gastrointestinal tract. This antigen is also in fetal gut and other fetal abdominal organs between 2–6 months of gestation. It can be found in the serum of carcinomatic patients and represents an extracellular product (5).

Recently, Coggin et al. (6) induced immunity to SV40-induced tumors in hamsters by injecting either irradiated hamster or mouse fetal tissue into the animals. In addition, Duff and Rapp (7) observed, in an indirect immunofluorescence test, that serum from pregnant hamsters stained the surface of SV40-transformed hamster cells.

This report enlarges on previous observations and compares surface antigens of one-celled unfertilized mouse eggs with those of mouse somatic cells transformed by SV40 or other oncogenic viruses, as well as with those of cells of other species transformed by SV40.

MATERIALS AND METHODS

Eggs.—Unfertilized mouse eggs were obtained from Swiss ICR mice according to the technique described in (1). Unfertilized hamster eggs were obtained from 6- to 8-week-old virgin Syrian female hamsters given intraperitoneal injections of serum gonadotropin (Equinex, Ayerst Lab. Inc., New York, N.Y.) at 0.4 IU/g of body weight, followed 2 days later with injection of chorionic gonadotropin (Pregnyl, Organon, W. Orange, N.J.) at 0.4 IU/g body weight. After 16 hours, the eggs were removed from the oviduct, and the cumulus oophorus and zona pellucida were removed by digestion with hyaluronidase and pronase, as described (1).

Somatic cells.—The following SV40-transformed cells were used: PF-1, of C57BL/6 mouse origin (1); S15, of strain A mouse origin (8); BTH, of Syrian hamster origin (obtained from Dr. A. J. Girardi, The Wistar Institute); GMK-Eva c12-A1, of African green monkey kidney origin (9); and WI26Va₄, of human origin. A polyoma virus-transformed mouse cell line, Py-Al/n, was received

22

through the kindness of Dr. Takemoto, National Institutes of Health, Bethesda, Maryland. A mouse cell line infected with Moloney leukemia virus, YAC, of strain A origin, was grown in ascites form (kindly provided by Dr. George Klein, Karolinska Institutet, Stockholm, Sweden). E1 and G1 cells derived from adenovirus 12-induced tumors in CBA mice, were procured from Dr. Leonard Berman, Mallory Institute of Pathology, Boston City Hospital, Boston, Massachusetts. The origin of MC57G mouse cells, induced by chemical carcinogen, was described (1). Thymus cells were obtained from 4-week-old C57BL/6 mice; spleen cells, from adult mice of the same strain.

Immunizations.—Guinea pigs (strain 13, Wistar colony) were immunized with unfertilized one-celled mouse eggs as described (1) to obtain anti egg (AE) serum. Guinea pigs were immunized with PF-1 and C57BL/6 spleen cells in 6 intracutaneous injections of 2×10^6 cells each in complete Freund's adjuvant (Difco catalog #0638-59).

C57BL/6 female mice were immunized against PF-1 cells in 6 intraperitoneal injections of cells suspended in phosphate-buffered saline. The first injection consisted of 5×10^4 cells and the remaining 5 injections, of 1×10^5 cells.

Cytotoxicity test.—The method used for one-celled mouse eggs and somatic cells was the same as that described in (1).

Colony inhibition test.—AE and anti-PF-1 guinea pig sera were absorbed by being mixed with 0.4 ml of a 1:10 dilution of immune serum with packed 1×10^7 cells. The mixture was maintained at room temperature for 1 hour and at 4°C for an additional hour; tubes were occasionally shaken. The colony inhibition test was performed with this serum, as described in (1).

RESULTS

Effect of AE Serum on Somatic Cells Transformed by Various Viruses

The results (table 1) indicate that AE serum shows the highest cytotoxic activity against SV40-

transformed S15 and PF-1 cells, somewhat less

TABLE 1.—Cytotoxic effect of AE guinea pig serum on mouse cells of various origins

Serum	Highest dilution of serum showing cyto-toxic effect against at least 50% of cells:				
	PF-1	S15	E1	YAC	Py-A1/n
Immune	1:96	1:96	1:12	1:24	1:12
Control	<1:3	<1:3	<1:3	<1:3	<1:3

activity against Moloney leukemia virus-infected YAC cells, and even less against adenovirus 12- (E1) and polyoma virus-transformed (Py-A1/n) cells.

Effect of AE Serum on SV40-Transformed Cells of Various Species Origin

The results in both the cytotoxicity and the colony inhibition tests (table 2) indicate that only the SV40-transformed PF-1 cells were susceptible to the cytotoxic effect of AE serum, whereas SV40-transformed cells of hamster, monkey, or human origin were not.

Absorption of Antibodies From AE Serum

AE sera were absorbed with cells of various origin and tested for their cytotoxic effect on mouse eggs. Only after absorption with the SV40-transformed S15 cells was the cytotoxicity titer of AE serum for eggs considerably reduced (table 3). Absorption of the AE serum with cells transformed by either polyoma or adenovirus had no effect on the cytotoxicity of the serum for eggs. Equally without effect was absorption of AE serum with Moloney virus-infected cells, malignant MC57G cells induced by chemical carcinogen, normal thymus cells, or SV40-transformed BTH cells.

24

TABLE 2.—Effect of AE guinea pig serum on SV40-transformed cells
of various species origin

| Cells | | Serum | Assays | |
Origin	Type		Colony inhibition*	Cytotoxicity †
Mouse	PF-1	I	3, 0, 9	1:96
		C	182, 185, 200	<1:3
Hamster	BTII	I	63, 67, 91	<1:3
		C	87, 53, 60	<1:3
Monkey	c12-A1	I	43, 37, 55	<1:3
		C	48, 39, 29	<1:3
Human	WI26Va₄	I	NT‡	<1:3
		C	NT	<1:3

*Number of colonies growing out of 300 cells seeded, for each of 3 petri dishes.
†Highest dilution of serum showing cytotoxic effect against at least 50% of cells.
‡NT: not tested.

Effect of Anti-PF-1 and Anti-Mouse Spleen Guinea Pig Serum on Mouse Eggs

Sera produced in guinea pigs against unfertilized one-celled mouse eggs were cytotoxic for mouse eggs and PF-1 cells; sera against PF-1 cells were cytotoxic for PF-1 cells and mouse eggs; sera against normal mouse spleen cells were cytotoxic for spleen cells and PF-1 cells only. Figures 1–3 show a typical cytotoxic reaction of unfertilized mouse eggs treated for 5–7 minutes with AE serum.

The results (table 4) indicate that the anti-C57BL/6 spleen serum, which showed much higher cytotoxicity for C57BL/6 spleen cells than for the SV40-transformed PF-1 cells, had no effect on mouse eggs. In contrast, the anti-PF-1 serum, which in dilutions of 1:48 and 1:24 was cytotoxic for PF-1 cells and normal spleen cells, respectively, was cytotoxic for mouse eggs at dilutions higher than 1:100.

The AE serum, not cytotoxic for spleen cells, was highly cytotoxic for PF-1 cells. The AE serum showed no cytotoxic effect on hamster eggs.

Lack of Cytotoxic Effect on Eggs of Anti-PF-1

Serum Produced in Syngeneic Mice

In contrast to the results obtained with anti-PF-1 guinea pig serum (table 4), serum obtained from C57BL/6 mice containing antibodies against PF-1 cells had little or no cytotoxic effect on mouse eggs. In the first test, only 2 of 23 eggs were destroyed after exposure to a 1:10 dilution of anti-PF-1 serum, whereas in the second test, none of the 29 eggs was damaged after exposure.

Absorption of Antibodies From Anti-PF-1 Guinea Pig Serum

The anti-PF-1 guinea pig serum was absorbed either with PF-1 cells or normal spleen cells and tested for its cytotoxic effect on cells. The results (table 5) indicate that absorption of anti-PF-1 serum with PF-1 cells completely eliminates its cytotoxic effect for any cells tested. In contrast, absorption of anti-PF-1 serum with mouse spleen cells does not reduce the cytotoxic effect of the serum for any cells tested, except for spleen cells.

DISCUSSION

The results of these experiments confirm those obtained previously (*1*), which indicates the species (mouse)-specificity of the AE serum. As with rat eggs (*1*), we failed to detect cytotoxic activity against hamster eggs in the AE serum. Similarly, the AE serum was not cytotoxic for hamster, human, or monkey cells transformed by SV40. It seems, therefore, that the antigen the mouse eggs have in common with the SV40-transformed cells is also species specific and that the SV40 "unmasked" early embryonic antigen is characteristic for each species, as indicated by cytotoxic tests with guinea pig antisera prepared against one-celled unfertilized mouse eggs emulsified in Freund's adjuvants. This antigen is apparently unrelated either to the structural or functional proteins of the virus itself, or to any "new" cellular antigens induced by infection with SV40. The species-specificity of the reaction could

TABLE 3.—Cytotoxicity of AE serum for mouse eggs after absorption of serum with cells of various origins

AE serum absorbed* with cells	Number of eggs destroyed after exposure to AE serum in dilution:				
	1:10	1:30	1:60	1:100	1:200
None	10/10	10/10	10/10	10/10	10/10
S15	10/10	9/10	0/10	0/10	NT
BTH	NT†	NT	8/9	NT	9/9
Py-Av/n	NT	NT	8/9	NT	9/9
YAC	NT	NT	9/9	NT	9/9
E1	NT	NT	9/9	NT	9/9
G1	NT	NT	8/9	NT	9/9
MC57G	10/10	9/10	10/10	7/10	NT
Thymus (C57BL/6)	NT	10/10	10/10	6/10	NT
Absorbed with various mouse organs‡	25/31	NT	NT	27/29	NT

*Sera were absorbed in dilution 1:10 with 10^7 cells/0.4 ml.
†NT: not tested.
‡This serum was absorbed by Dr. L. J. Old with various organs of inbred mice representing all major *H-2* locus-controlled antigens.

Table 4.—Comparative effects of AE, anti-PF-1, and anti-mouse-spleen guinea pig sera on eggs, PF-1, and spleen cells

Serum	Highest dilution of serum showing cytotoxic effect against at least 50% of cells			
	PF-1	Spleen	Mouse eggs	Hamster eggs
Anti-spleen	1:24	1:512	<1:3	NT*
AE	1:96	<1:10	>1:120	<1:3
Anti-PF-1	1:48	1:24	>1:100	NT

*NT: not tested.

Table 5.—Cytotoxic effect of anti-PF-1 serum absorbed with PF-1 or mouse-spleen cells on SV40-transformed cells

Anti-PF-1 serum absorbed with cells	Highest dilution of serum showing cytotoxic effect against at least 50% of cells				
	PF-1	BTII	c12-A1	Mouse spleen	Mouse egg
None	1:48	1:12	1:24	1:96	>1:100
C57BL/6 spleen	1:48	1:12	1:24	<1:10	>1:100
PF-1	<1:10	<1:10	<1:10	<1:10	<1:10
Normal guinea pig serum	<1:3	<1:3	<1:3	<1:3	<1:3

be checked easily in experiments on cross-reactivity between immune serum produced against eggs of species other than mice and SV40-transformed cells of homologous species.

Whether infection or transformation by SV40, or both, represents a unique system of "unmasking" early embryonic antigens is difficult to decide at present. In contrast to the titers obtained with cells transformed by SV40, AE serum was cytotoxic for mouse cells transformed by either polyoma virus or adenovirus only at a very low dilution. Moreover, in the absorption tests, the cytotoxic activity of AE serum for eggs was removed by absorption of the serum with SV40-transformed mouse cells, but not with cells transformed by the other viruses. Why the absorption failed is under investigation. The failure may have been caused by quantitative differences in embryo antigens unmasked by different viruses. In other words, with more cells for absorption and/or further dilution of the sera, some absorbing activity might be observed. This is very unlikely, as the titer of 200 is practically the endpoint of cytotoxic activity of AE sera against mouse eggs. More probably, different embryo antigens are unmasked by different viruses. Otherwise, cross-reactivity among various virus-induced tumors would be more common. A cross-reactivity between antigens in polyoma-transformed hamster cells and hamster cells derived from a 12-day embryo was described by Pearson and Freeman (11). On the other hand, Ting (12) was unable to induce resistance to polyoma tumors in mice after immunization with syngeneic mouse-embryo tissue. The problem remains open for investigation, particularly in relation to the antigens present in embryos at stages of development later than the one-celled stage.

Mouse serum containing antibodies against syngeneic SV40-transformed cells was not cytotoxic for mouse eggs, whereas serum produced in guinea pigs against the same cells was. Another reason may be that the mouse egg does not contain SV40 tumor-specific transplantation antigen (TSTA).

Antibodies against mouse egg are not toxic for other species of SV40-transformed cells, and antibodies against TSTA are not toxic for mouse eggs. Failure of the mouse serum to react may, perhaps, be explained by the natural tolerance of the animal to the embryo antigen present in the one-celled egg. On the other hand, the embryo antigen of mouse eggs may represent an antigen immunogenic for guinea pigs, but haptenic for mice.

The ability of the hamster to react against SV40-transformed syngeneic cells after immunization with hamster embryo cells (6) makes this system different from the SV40-mouse egg system. The immunogenic reactivity of the hamster might be explained by the fact that 9- and 12-day hamster embryos were used for immunization. Older mouse embryos might also differ immunogenically and immunosensitively from one-celled unfertilized eggs. In light of the negative results obtained in cross-reactivity tests between AE serum and adult mouse tissue (spleen) on the one hand, and anti-spleen serum and mouse eggs on the other, it will be interesting to determine when, in the prenatal or postnatal period, the reactivity of the tissues against AE serum becomes suppressed.

Considering the fact that a) AE serum is not toxic for SV40-transformed cells of other species, b) guinea pig anti-PF-1(SV40-transformed cells) serum is cytotoxic for SV40-transformed cells of *other* species in addition to the mouse, and c) absorption of guinea pig anti-PF-1 serum with normal spleen cells does not affect its cytotoxicity for SV40-transformed cells, we may postulate the existence of at least two types of antigens in SV40-transformed cells. One type, probably coded by the virus itself, causes resistance to syngeneic challenge with tumor cells and may be involved in the interspecies cross-reactivity between various cell lines transformed by SV40. The other type represents an early embryonic antigen repressed during growth and differentiation of the organism and derepressed by infection and transformation of the cells by SV40. Whether other oncogenic viruses may unmask other embryonic antigens of the mouse and of other species is a question for a study in itself.

REFERENCES

(1) BARANSKA W, KOLDOVSKY P, KOPROWSKI H: Antigenic study of unfertilized mouse eggs: Crossreactivity with SV40-induced antigens. Proc Nat Acad Sci USA 67:193–199, 1970

(2) BUTTLE GA, EPERON JL, KOVACS E: An antigen in malignant and in embryonic tissues. Nature (London) 194:780, 1962

(3) ABELEV GI, PEROVA SD, KHRAMKOVA NI, et al: Production of embryonal α-globulin by transplantable mouse hepatomas. Transplantation 1:174–180, 1963

(4) GOLD P, FREEDMAN SO: Demonstration of tumorspecific antigens in human colonic carcinomata by immunological tolerance and absorption techniques. J Exp Med 121:439 462, 1965

(5) GOLD P, KRUPEY J, ANSARI H: Position of the carcinoembryonic antigen of the human digestive system in ultrastructure of tumor cell surface. J Nat Cancer Inst 45:219–225, 1970

(6) COGGIN JH, AMBROSE KR, ANDERSON NG: Fetal antigen capable of inducing transplantation immunity against SV40 hamster tumor cells. J Immun 105:524–526, 1970

(7) DUFF R, RAPP F: Reaction of serum from pregnant hamsters with surface of cells transformed by SV40. J Immun 105:521–523, 1970

(8) KOLDOVSKY P, JENSEN F: In preparation.

(9) KOPROWSKI H, JENSEN FC, STEPLEWSKI Z: Activation of production of infectious tumor virus SV40 in heterokaryon cultures. Proc Nat Acad Sci USA 58:127–133, 1967

(10) JENSEN F, KOPROWSKI H, PONTÉN JA: Rapid transformation of human fibroblast cultures by Simian virus 40. Proc Nat Acad Sci USA 50:343–348, 1963

(11) PEARSON G, FREEMAN G: Evidence suggesting a relationship between polyoma virus-induced transplantation antigen and normal embryonic antigen. Cancer Res 28:1665–1673, 1968

(12) TING RC: Failure to induce transplantation resistance against polyoma tumour cells with syngeneic embryonic tissues. Nature (London) 217:858–859, 1968.

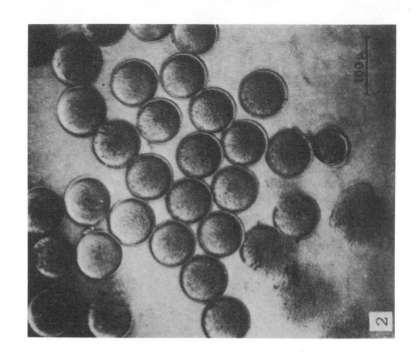

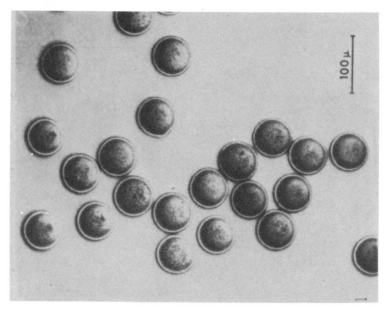

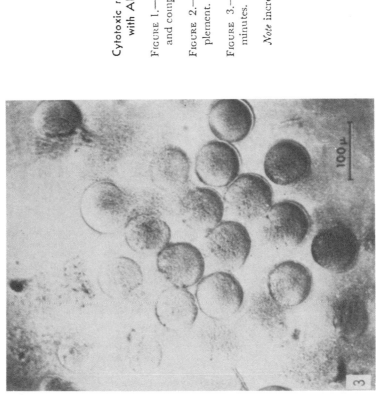

Cytotoxic reaction of unfertilized one-celled mouse eggs treated with AE guinea pig serum in the presence of complement.

FIGURE 1.—Eggs treated for 1 hour with control guinea pig serum and complement.

FIGURE 2.—Eggs treated for 5 minutes with AE serum and complement.

FIGURE 3.—Eggs treated with AE serum and complement for 7 minutes.

Note increase with time of number of cells destroyed.

Inactivation of T Antigen-Forming Capacities of Simian Virus 40 and Adenovirus 12 by Ultraviolet Irradiation

HIROSHI YAMAMOTO AND HIROTO SHIMOJO

The transforming capacities of polyoma virus and adenovirus are more resistant to inactivation by irradiation than are their infectivities, suggesting that the target sizes of the genome required for transformation may be smaller than those which are essential for viral replication (2, 4, 6, 8, 9, 13). In accord with these findings, it has been reported that the capacities of simian virus 40 (SV40) and adenovirus 12 (Ad12) to induce T antigen were more resistant to inactivation by irradiation than their infectivities (4, 7, 8, 11, 13, 19). However, zur Hausen (23) reported that the infectivity and T antigen-forming capacity of Ad12 were inactivated at the same rate by ultraviolet (UV) irradiation. Strohl (19) reported that T antigen-forming capacity of Ad12 was a little more resistant to UV inactivation than infectivity.

The present communication describes the UV inactivation of T antigen-forming capacities of SV40 and Ad12, showing that the capacities were inactivated at the same rate as their infectivities when the capacity was measured in nongrowing cells and that T-antigen formation was enhanced in cells multiply infected and in cells in a growing state. Reasons for the discrepancies among reports hitherto published are discussed.

MATERIALS AND METHODS

Cell cultures and viruses. Primary or secondary cultures of green monkey kidney cells (GMK) and human embryonic kidney cells (HEK) were used for SV40 and Ad12, respectively. SV40 Conn II strain, which was isolated in this laboratory, and Ad12 Huie strain were used. Crude virus fluid was prepared by sonic treatment of suspensions of cells showing cytopathic effect in Eagle's minimal essential medium (MEM) without serum and by centrifugation at 3,000 rev/min ($1,500 \times g$) for 30 min. The infectivity of virus was titrated by plaque assay in GMK and HEK as described (22) and expressed in plaque-forming units (PFU).

Preparation of SV40 DNA. The purification of SV40 virions and the extraction of deoxyribonucleic acid (DNA) therefrom were carried out in a similar manner to that applied to adenovirus (18). Virions were purified by isopycnic sedimentation in CsCl solution, and DNA was extracted from the purified virions (density 1.34) by treatment with sodium dodecyl sulfate (0.5%) and phenol extraction. Phenol extraction was repeated, and the final aqueous layer containing DNA was dialyzed against phosphate-buffered saline (PBS).

Inactivation of virus by UV irradiation. A 1-ml amount of virus stock was spread in a thin layer in a petri dish (10 cm in diameter) and irradiated by a germicidal lamp (10 w) at a distance of 30 cm for the time indicated in results. Water lost by evaporation during irradiation was replaced by sterile water, which was used to rinse the dish after irradiation. Although irradiation was carried out mostly with crude virus fluid, it was confirmed that the same inactivation kinetics as that with virions purified by isopycnic sedimentation in CsCl solution (density 1.34) could be obtained, possibly due to the absence of serum in the suspending medium.

34

Measurement of the T antigen-forming capacity. T antigen-forming units (TFU) described by Uchida et al. (21) to measure the capacity of SV40 to induce T antigen were used with a technical modification. Details of the immunofluorescence technique to examine Ad12 T antigen have been described (17). Narrow-reacting serum was used to avoid the involvement of virion antigens. The same technique was used to stain SV40 T antigen with anti-SV40 T conjugate prepared from sera of hamsters transplanted with SV40 tumors. It was confirmed that these sera did not contain antibody against SV40 virion antigen. A monolayer of GMK or HEK on a cover slip was inoculated with 0.2 ml of fourfold serial dilutions of virus. After adsorption at 36 C for 2 hr, the cover slips were incubated at 36 C for 72 hr (SV40) or 48 hr (Ad12 and SV40 DNA) in Eagle's MEM containing cytosine arabinoside (AraC, 10 μg per ml) to avoid secondary infection. The cover slips were rinsed in PBS, dried, treated with CCl₄, and stained. The numbers of cells with and without specific fluorescence were counted under a fluorescence microscope. Preparations in which less than 10% of cells showed specific fluorescence were selected and used for the calculation of TFU for the reason described below. Two to three preparations were used for the determination of TFU. Microscopic observation at a high magnification was necessary for Ad12 so as not to miss faint fluorescent flecks. Therefore, TFU of Ad12 were calculated by the percentage of T antigen-positive cells among the cells on a cover slip. The original method of Uchida et al. (21) was also used, in which 80 to 100 neutralizing units of rabbit antiserum, instead of AraC, was added to avoid the secondary infection. Induction of T antigen in growing cells was examined as follows. After adsorption of virus for 2 hr, cells were resuspended, diluted 10 times in growth medium containing 80 to 100 neutralizing units of anti-SV40 serum, and plated onto cover slips in small bottles. After incubation for the indicated time, T antigen-positive cells were examined. TFU were calculated by the number of T antigen-positive cells at each dilution.

Determination of PFU and TFU of SV40 DNA. PFU and TFU of SV40 DNA were measured by the method of McCutchan and Pagano (15). GMK monolayers were washed twice with a mixture of Eagle's MEM and PBS in equal amounts, containing neither antibiotics nor sodium bicarbonate. A 0.2-ml amount of DNA, diluted with the same medium containing diethylaminoethyl dextran (Pharmacia, Uppsala; molecular weight, 3 × 10⁶) at a concentration of 500 μg/ml, was inoculated in a bottle or on a cover slip. After adsorption at room temperature for 30 min, cells were washed with Eagle's MEM. Further procedures were the same as described above.

RESULTS

Time course of T-antigen synthesis. Time course of T-antigen synthesis by UV-irradiated or unirradiated SV40 and Ad12 was tested. The appearance of T antigen-positive cells was slower in cultures infected with UV-irradiated SV40 and Ad12 than with unirradiated virus. Percentage of T antigen-positive cells in GMK infected with UV-irradiated and unirradiated SV40 increased up to 72 hr postinfection (pi) and then remained unchanged. Therefore, 72 hr pi was adopted as the time to examine SV40 T antigen. Percentage of T antigen-positive cells in HEK infected with UV-irradiated and unirradiated Ad12 increased up to 48 hr; thus, 48 hr pi was adopted as the time to examine Ad12 T antigen. Forty-eight hours pi was adopted as the time to examine T antigen induced by SV40 DNA, since the decrease in the percentage of T antigen-positive cells was observed from 48 to 72 hr pi.

Dose response of T antigen-forming capacity. The relationship between the percentages of T antigen-positive cells and the dilutions of virus is shown in Fig. 1 and 2. A linear relationship was always observed in repeated experiments when the percentage of T antigen-positive cells was less than 10%. The responses deviated from the linear relationship in the range in which more cells showed specific fluorescence. When similar tests were carried out with UV-irradiated SV40 and Ad12, the percentage of T antigen-positive cells was obtained as expected by virus dilution in the range in which less than a few per cent of cells showed specific fluorescence. In contrast to the unirradiated virus, UV-irradiated SV40 and Ad12 induced T antigen in more cells than expected when cells were infected with lower dilutions of

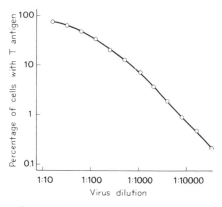

FIG. 1. *Dose-response curve of T antigen-forming capacity of Ad12. HEK cells on a cover slip, infected with twofold serial dilutions of Ad12 virus, were incubated at 36 C for 48 hr in medium containing AraC. Cells were stained as described. The percentages of cells with specific fluorescence were counted under a fluorescence microscope.*

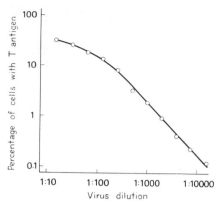

FIG. 2. *Dose-response curve of T antigen-forming capacity of SV40. GMK cells were infected with SV40 and expressed in the same manner as in Fig. 1.*

TABLE 1. *Induction of T antigen by UV-irradiated Ad12 and SV40*[a]

Inocula		Percentage of cells with T antigen		Ratio (O/E)
Virus	Dilution	Observed value (O)	Expected value (E)[b]	
		%	%	
Ad12 (UV-irradiated for 15 min)	1:1	71.7	21.76	3.29
	1:2	28.6	10.88	2.62
	1:4	10.7	5.44	1.97
	1:8	4.1	2.72	1.50
	1:16	1.35	1.36	0.99
	1:32	0.68	0.68	1.00
SV40 (UV-irradiated for 27 min)	1:1	18.8	6.56	2.87
	1:2	5.9	3.28	1.80
	1:4	1.43	1.64	0.87
	1:8	0.68	0.82	0.83
	1:16	0.41	0.41	1.00

[a] HEK or GMK, on a cover slip, infected with UV-irradiated Ad12 or SV40, was maintained in medium containing AraC. After incubation at 36 C for 48 hr (Ad12) or 72 hr (SV40), T antigen in cells was stained. The number of cells with T antigen was counted under a fluorescence microscope, and the percentage of cells with T antigen was calculated. The standard deviation was approximately ±15% of the observed value at each dilution.

[b] The expected value was calculated from the percentage of T antigen-positive cells at the highest dilution in the table.

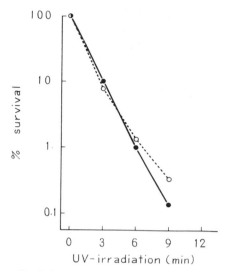

FIG. 3. *Inactivation of Ad12 PFU and TFU by UV irradiation. After UV irradiation of Ad12 for the time indicated, PFU and TFU were measured. Survivals of PFU (●) and TFU (○) relative to unirradiated control are depicted.*

virus (Table 1), suggesting that multiplicity reactivation may have occurred in cells infected with UV-irradiated virus at a higher multiplicity.

A linear dose response of SV40 DNA, unirradiated and UV-irradiated for 6 min, was observed in the range in which less than 0.5% of cells were T antigen-positive. The dose response of SV40 DNA, UV-irradiated for 12 min, could not be confirmed. Therefore, TFU of SV40 DNA, UV-irradiated for 12 min, were calculated from preparations which showed less than 10 T antigen-positive cells in the whole area.

Inactivation of SV40 and Ad12 in PFU and TFU. The rate of inactivation of PFU and TFU of SV40 or Ad12 after UV irradiation is shown in Fig. 3 and 4. PFU and TFU of SV40 or Ad12 were inactivated at the same rate, roughly following a single-hit curve. The relative survivals of SV40 DNA in terms of PFU and TFU are shown in Fig. 5. PFU and TFU of SV40 DNA were inactivated at the same rate, in accord with the UV inactivation of SV40 virions. This observation indicates that UV inactivation of virions resulted from damage to DNA and not by other factors, such as inefficient adsorption or uncoating of irradiated virions.

Formation of T antigen in growing cells. Secondary cultures of GMK monolayers were in-

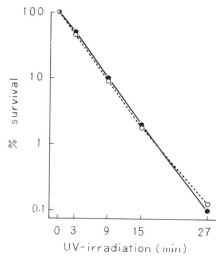

FIG. 4. *Inactivation of SV40 PFU and TFU by UV irradiation. Procedure and symbols as if .... in Fig. 3.*

fected with SV40 that had been UV-irradiated for 22 and 45 min (reduction of PFU about 10^{-2} and 10^{-5}, respectively). After adsorption, cells were subcultured on a cover slip and incubated at 36 C in a CO_2 incubator. T antigen-positive cells were examined at 72, 96, and 120 hr pi. Aggregates of more than 2 T antigen-positive cells appeared 96 hr pi, possibly due to cell-to-cell infection in medium containing antiserum. Therefore, an aggregate was counted as a T antigen-positive cell. At the same time, PFU and TFU (in media containing either AraC or antiserum) were measured (Table 2). As shown in the table, T antigen-positive cells increased in growing cultures, suggesting that T-antigen formation by UV-irradiated SV40 may have been enhanced in growing cells. It was noticed that TFU measured in media containing antiserum gave a slightly higher value than that in media containing AraC. A similar test was carried out with HEK cells, infected with Ad12, unirradiated and UV-irradiated for 10 min. However, TFU of UV-irradiated Ad12 in growing cells gave variable results and are not included in the table. It was also confirmed that TFU measured in media containing antiserum gave a slightly higher value than those in media containing AraC.

Then, semiconfluent monolayers of HEK were infected with Ad12, UV-irradiated for 15 min. After adsorption, half of the cultures were maintained in growth medium containing antiserum, and the other half was maintained in the same medium containing AraC instead of antiserum and incubated at 36 C. The numbers of cells in cultures and the percentages of T antigen-positive cells were counted at the times indicated (Fig. 6). It was shown that T antigen-positive cells increased in parallel with the growth of cells. Thus, it was suggested that the induction of T antigen may be enhanced in growing cells.

DISCUSSION

PFU are calculated from the number of plaques produced by diluted virus under conditions in which it is improbable for a single cell to receive more than one virion. To compare PFU to the other biological capacities of viruses, measurements must be made under the same condition. Thus, TFU titration described by Uchida et al. (21) was measured with a modified method in which AraC was used instead of antiserum. Examination of the incorporation of ^{3}H-thymidine in autoradiograms confirmed that DNA synthesis, either cellular or viral, was completely inhibited in cells maintained in media containing AraC and no serum. Thus, cells were maintained in a nongrowing state, and the secondary infection by replicating virus was prevented.

The measurement of TFU in medium con-

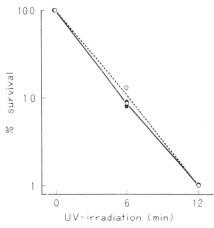

FIG. 5. *Inactivation of SV40 DNA PFU and TFU by UV irradiation. SV40 DNA was irradiated by UV in the same manner as virus for 6 and 12 min. After irradiation, PFU and TFU of unirradiated DNA and UV-irradiated DNA were determined. Survivals of PFU (●) and TFU (○) relative to the unirradiated control are depicted.*

37

TABLE 2. *Induction of T antigen in cells under various conditions*[a]

Determination	Unirradiated	UV irradiated[b]		Titer reduction	
		A	B	A	B
SV40					
PFU	$10^{7.2}$	$10^{5.0}$	$10^{2.1}$	$10^{-2.2}$	$10^{-5.1}$
TFU (AraC)[c]	$10^{7.5}$	$10^{5.1}$	$10^{2.7}$	$10^{-2.4}$	$10^{-4.8}$
TFU (antiserum)[c]	$10^{7.3}$	NT[d]	$10^{3.2}$	NT	$10^{-4.1}$
TFU in growing cells					
72 hr pi	$10^{7.4}$	$10^{5.6}$	$10^{3.8}$	$10^{-1.8}$	$10^{-3.6}$
96 hr pi	$10^{7.6}$	$10^{6.2}$	$10^{4.4}$	$10^{-1.1}$	$10^{-3.2}$
120 hr pi	$10^{7.6}$	NT	$10^{4.4}$	NT	$10^{-3.2}$
Ad12					
PFU	$10^{6.0}$	$10^{3.0}$		$10^{-3.0}$	
TFU (AraC)[c]	$10^{6.5}$	$10^{3.7}$		$10^{-2.7}$	
TFU (antiserum)[c]	$10^{6.1}$	$10^{5.0}$		$10^{-1.1}$	

[a] GMK or HEK were infected with SV40 or Ad12, respectively; PFU and TFU were determined as described in text and expressed in PFU or TFU per 0.2 ml.

[b] UV irradiation of SV40 for 22 min (A) and 45 min (B) and of Ad12 for 10 min.

[c] Measured in cells maintained in media containing AraC. Measured in cells maintained in media containing 80 to 100 neutralizing units of antiserum.

[d] Not tested.

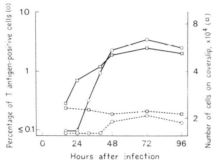

FIG. 6. *Time course of T-antigen synthesis by UV-irradiated Ad12. After infection of semiconfluent monolayers of HEK with Ad12 UV-irradiated for 15 min, the cultures were incubated in media containing either AraC or antiserum. T antigen-positive cells were examined at the indicated time. At the same time, the number of cells on a cover slip was measured. Solid lines represent the percentage of T antigen-positive cells (○) and the number of growing cells maintained in media containing antiserum on a cover slip (□). Broken lines show the percentage of T antigen-positive cells (○) and the number of nongrowing cells in media containing AraC on a cover slip (□).*

taining AraC became feasible, since a linear relationship between the number of T antigen-positive cells and virus dilutions was confirmed in cells inoculated with diluted virus. Deviations from the linear dose response were observed when cells were infected at higher multiplicities,

probably due to Poisson distribution of unirradiated virions and to multiplicity reactivation of UV-irradiated virions.

PFU and TFU of SV40 or Ad12 were inactivated at the same rate, roughly following a single-hit curve. A similar result was obtained when Ad12 was inactivated by electron beam irradiation, although the inactivation curve deviated somewhat from a single-hit curve (data are not included). Although the present results and those reported by zur Hausen (23) showed the same inactivation rate of the capacity to induce T antigen and the infectivity by UV irradiation, many investigators have reported that the former is far more resistant than the latter (5, 7, 8, 11). However, in these studies (5, 7, 8, 11), the capacity to induce T antigen was measured in the range in which more than 10% of cells induced T antigen. The present study suggested that multiplicity reactivation of irradiated virus in T-antigen formation may have occurred in cells in which more than a few per cent of cells became T antigen-positive. It is, therefore, suggested that the marked difference in sensitivity to UV inactivation suggested between plaque-forming and T antigen-forming capacities in other reports (5, 7, 8, 11) may be due to multiplicity reactivation. The multiplicity reactivation of UV-irradiated SV40 and Ad12 was also confirmed in studies of plaque-forming and infective center-forming capacities (Yamamoto, *unpublished data*).

Strohl (19) reported that T antigen-forming capacity of Ad12 was a little more resistant to UV inactivation than infectivity. Uchida (*per-*

sonal communication) also obtained a similar result with SV40. In these studies, T antigen-forming capacity was measured under conditions in which multiplicity reactivation could be ruled out. However, cells were maintained in media without AraC, and a small portion of cells could grow, in which T antigen-formation may be enhanced. Thus, it is conceivable that the measurement of T antigen-forming capacity may vary, depending upon the experimental conditions employed. At one extreme, TFU may be equal to PFU in nongrowing cells, such as cells maintained in media containing AraC. On the other hand, T antigen-forming capacity may be four times more resistant than infectivity when measured by transformation (22). Measurement of TFU in growing cells and in cells maintained in media containing antiserum should result in values between the two extremes (Fig. 7), and discrepancies among reports may be due to reactivation of irradiated virus in cells multiply infected and to the enhancement of T-antigen formation in growing cells.

The UV inactivation of Ad12 or SV40 PFU and TFU activity was due neither to inefficient adsorption nor to uncoating of UV-irradiated virions but may have resulted from damage to viral DNA induced by UV irradiation, since PFU and TFU of SV40 DNA were inactivated at the same rate. It is suggested that similar damage to Ad12 DNA can be induced by UV irradiation, since UV-irradiated Ad5 was uncoated at the same rate as the unirradiated control (14). The above observation, however, cannot be interpreted to show the relative target size of genome loci responsible for the induction of T antigen, since many observations indicate that the gene for T antigen synthesis must be a part of the whole viral genome. Especially, estimation of the portion of the viral genome transcribed in SV40 or Ad2-transformed cells (1, 10, 16) clearly showed that the gene for T antigen is only a part of the viral genome. In accord with these estimations, the gene for transformation by SV40 was estimated to be about one-fourth of the whole viral genome by UV inactivation and that for tumor-production of Ad12 was 5 to 7% of the viral genome; all the transformed cells were T antigen-positive (22).

It has been suggested that T-antigen formation may be enhanced in growing cells. Ben-Bassat et al. demonstrated that the synthesis of T antigen was enhanced in replicating 3T3 cells infected with SV40 (3). The presence of AraC in medium that inhibited cellular DNA synthesis may contribute to the inefficient formation of T antigen and may have resulted in the same rate of UV inactivation in PFU and TFU. Although mul-

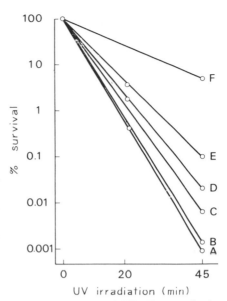

FIG. 7. *Inactivation of SV40 T antigen-forming capacity by UV irradiation, measured under various conditions. After UV irradiation of SV40 for the time indicated, TFU were measured under various conditions, and survival relative to unirradiated control is depicted. Inactivation of (A) PFU, (B) TFU in AraC, (C) TFU in antiserum, (D) TFU in growing cells measured at 72 hr pi, or (E) TFU in growing cells measured at 96 hr pi. (F) UV inactivation curve of transforming capacity of SV40, as described elsewhere (22).*

tiplicity reactivation and enhancement of T-antigen formation in growing cells were only suggested and could not be completely proven, it was concluded that the size of the gene for T antigen could not be estimated by UV inactivation.

LITERATURE CITED

1. Aloni, Y., E. Winocour, and L. Sachs. 1968. Characterization of the simian virus 40-specific RNA in virus-yielding and transformed cells. J. Mol. Biol. 31:415–429.
2. Basilico, C., and G. di Mayorka. 1965. Radiation target size of the lytic and transforming ability of polyoma virus. Proc. Nat. Acad. Sci. U.S.A. 54:125–127.
3. Ben-Bassat, H., M. Inbar, and L. Sachs. 1970. Requirement for cell replication after SV40 infection for a structural change of the cell surface membrane. Virology 40:854–859.
4. Benjamin, T. L. 1965. Relative target sizes for the inactivation of the transforming and reproductive ability of polyoma virus. Proc. Nat. Acad. U.S.A. 54:121–124.
5. Carp, R. I., and R. M. Gilden. 1965. The inactivation of simian virus 40 infectivity and antigen-inducing capacity by ultraviolet light. Virology 27:639–641.
6. Casto, B. C. 1968. Effects of ultraviolet irradiation on the transforming and plaque-forming capacities of simian adenovirus SA7. J. Virol. 2:641–642.

7. Coppey, J., and R. Wicker. 1968. Inactivation par les radiations U.V., X et gamma de deux propriétés du virus SV-40: infectivité et induction de l'antigène nucléaire précoce. Ann. Inst. Pasteur 115:478–485.

8. Defendi, V., F. Jensen, and G. Sauer. 1967. Analysis of some viral function related to neoplastic transformation, p. 645–662. In J. S. Colter and W. Paranchych (ed.), The molecular biology of viruses, Academic Press Inc., New York.

9. Finkelstein, J. Z., and R. M. McAllister. 1969. Ultraviolet inactivation of the cytocydal and transforming activities of human adenovirus type 1. J. Virol. 3:353–354.

10. Fujinaga, K., and M. Green. 1970. The mechanism of viral carcinogenesis by DNA mammalian viruses. VII. Viral genes transcribed in adenovirus type 2 infected and transformed cells. Proc. Nat. Acad. Sci. U.S.A. 65:375–385.

11. Gilead, Z., and H. S. Ginsberg. 1966. Comparison of the rates of ultraviolet inactivation of the capacity of type 12 adenovirus to infect cells and to induce T antigen formation. J. Bacteriol. 92:1853–1854.

12. Ginosa, W. 1968. Inactivation of viruses by ionizing radiation and by heat, p. 139–210. In K. Maramorosh and H. Koprowski (ed.), Methods in virology, vol. 4. Academic Press Inc., New York.

13. Latarjet, R., R. Cramer, and L. Montagier. 1967. Inactivation by UV-, X- and γ-radiation, of the infecting and transforming capacities of polyoma virus. Virology 33:104–111.

14. Lawrence, W. C., and H. S. Ginsberg. 1967. Intracellular uncoating of type 5 adenovirus deoxyribonucleic acid. J. Virol. 1:851–867.

15. McCutchan, J. H., and J. S. Pagano. 1968. Enhancement of the infectivity of simian virus 40 deoxyribonucleic acid with diethylaminoethyl-dextran. J. Nat. Cancer Inst. 41: 351–357.

16. Oda, K., and R. Dulbecco. 1968. Regulation of transcription of the SV40 DNA in productively infected and in transformed cells. Proc. Nat. Acad. Sci. U.S.A. 60:525–532.

17. Shimojo, H., H. Yamamoto, and C. Abe. 1967. Differentiation of adenovirus 12 antigens in cultured cells with immunofluorescent analysis. Virology 31:748–752.

18. Shimojo, H., and T. Yamashita. 1968. Induction of DNA synthesis by adenoviruses in contact-inhibited hamster cells. Virology 36:422–433.

19. Strohl, W. A. 1969. The response of BHK 21 cells to infection with type 12 adenovirus I. Cell killing and T antigen synthesis as correlated viral genome function. Virology 39:642–652.

20. Uchida, S., S. Watanabe, and M. Kato. 1966. Incomplete growth of simian virus 40 in African green monkey kidney cultures induced by serial undiluted passages. Virology 28:135–141.

21. Uchida, S., K. Yoshiike, S. Watanabe, and A. Furuno. 1968. Antigen-forming defective viruses of simian virus 40. Virology 34:1–8.

22. Yamamoto, H. 1970. Inactivation of the transforming capacity of SV40 and the oncogenicity of adenovirus 12 by ultraviolet irradiation. Jap. J. Microbiol. 14:487–493.

23. zur Hausen, H. 1967. Induction of specific chromosomal aberrations by adenovirus type 12 in human embryonic kidney cells. J. Virol. 1:1174–1185.

40

Ronald Duff
Fred Rapp
Janet S. Butel

Transformation of Hamster Cells by Variants of PARA- Adenovirus 7 Able to Induce SV40 Tumor Antigen in the Cytoplasm

Hamster embryo fibroblasts (HEF) are transformed *in vitro* by the PARA (defective SV40)-adenovirus 7 (ad 7) hybrid virus (*1*). The normal localization of the SV40 tumor (T) antigen in PARA transformed HEF cells as well as in productively infected green monkey kidney (GMK) cells is in the nucleus; however, the isolation of T antigen variants from a PARA-ad 7 stock has recently been reported (*2*). These variants are characterized by the appearance of the SV40 T antigen in the cytoplasm of infected GMK cells. Other characteristics of these cytoplasmic variants of PARA closely resemble those described for the parental SP2 stock of PARA-ad 7. The T antigen located in the cytoplasm during the replicative cycle of these variants in GMK cells is serologically similar or identical to the T antigen localized in the nucleus of GMK cells following infection with SV40 or the parental PARA-ad 7 (*2*). Other workers have also recently reported cytoplasmic localization of papovavirus-induced antigens (*3*, *4*). This report describes transformation of hamster embryo fibroblasts (HEF) by the cytoplasmic variants of PARA and some of the characteristics of the transformed cells.

Separate cultures of HEF were exposed to one of the three strains of the cytoplasmic PARA-ad 7 variants (1cT, 2cT, 3cT). The method used has been described previously (*1*). One milliliter of a virus-containing dilution was adsorbed with 8×10^5 cells in suspension for 3 hours. The cells were then placed into 60-mm petri dishes and grown in Eagle's basal medium (CaCl$_2$ concentration reduced to 0.1 m*M*), 10% fetal calf serum, 10% tryptose phosphate broth and 0.2% NaHCO$_3$. Seventeen days after virus infection, the cultures were stained with Wright's stain and transformed foci counted microscopically. Comparison of the transforming frequency of HEF by variants 1cT,

2cT, 3cT and the parental SP2 virus is presented in Table 1. The cytoplasmic variants transformed HEF at a frequency which was significantly lower than transformation induced by the parental SP2 stock of PARA-ad 7. However, among the cytoplasmic variants, 2cT transformed HEF at a frequency which was about three to six times greater than the cytoplasmic PARA-ad 7 variants.

HEF which have been transformed by SP2 always contain nuclear SV40 T antigen when examined by fluorescent antibody techniques (*5*). Cells transformed *in vitro* by 2cT were examined to determine the localization of the SV40 T antigen within the cells. A single 2cT-transformed focus of HEF was isolated and grown into a cell line (2cT-1). These cells were morphologically similar to the cuboidal type which have been described for hamster cells transformed by other variants of PARA which induce nuclear localization of SV40 T antigen. When examined at passage ten for the localization of the SV40 T antigen by indirect immunofluorescence, a large majority of the transformed cells were found to contain the SV40 T antigen in the cytoplasm. However, a small proportion of the cells contained nuclear T antigen.

The oncogenic potential of the 2cT-1 cell line was established by injecting 10^5 cells subcutaneously into weanling Syrian hamsters (Con Olsen). After a latent period ranging from 6 to 11 weeks, the transformed cells induced tumors in 6 of 17 hamsters. The tumors were removed from the animals and grown in cell culture to determine the localization of the SV40 T antigen. This antigen was found to be in the cytoplasm of the cells from five of the six tumors during the early passages (passage 1 through 3). The remaining tumor was a mixture of cytoplasmic T positive and nuclear T positive cells. Sera from these tumor-bearing

TABLE 1

Transformation of Hamster Embryo Fibroblasts by Cytoplasmic PARA Variants and Parental PARA (SP2) Virus

Virus	Virus dilution	PFU/plate[a]	FFU/plate[b, c]	FFU:PFU
PARA (1cT)[d]	1:10	3.0×10^5	3.00	1:100,000
	1:20	1.5×10^5	1.30	1:115,385
	1:40	7.5×10^4	0.50	1:150,000
PARA (2cT)[d]	1:10	2.0×10^5	7.00	1:28,571
	1:20	1.0×10^5	3.50	1:28,571
	1:40	5.0×10^4	1.50	1:33,333
PARA (3cT)[d]	1:10	4.0×10^5	2.30	1:173,913
	1:20	2.0×10^5	1.25	1:160,000
	1:40	1.0×10^5	0.50	1:200,000
PARA (SP2)	1:10	2.0×10^4	36.25	1:552
	1:20	1.0×10^4	19.50	1:513
	1:40	5.0×10^3	10.25	1:488

[a] PFU, Plaque-forming units as determined by plaque formation in GMK cells, preinfected with helper adenovirus 7; based on average of 4 plates per dilution.

[b] Average of 4 plates per dilution.

[c] FFU, Focus-forming units, determined by transformation of hamster embryo fibroblasts.

[d] Cytoplasmic PARA variants.

TABLE 2

Oncogenic Characteristics of Cell Clones Following Transformation by a PARA Cytoplasmic Variant

Clone	T Antigen localization[a]	Number of hamsters injected[b]	Number of hamsters with tumors	Latent period (weeks)
2cT-1a	Cytoplasm	10	10	3–4
2cT-1b	Nuclear	10	6	8–14

[a] Cells were tested for SV40 T antigen by the indirect fluorescent technique.

[b] 10^5 cells were injected following 5 passages after cloning.

animals contained antibodies which reacted with both the SV40 T antigen in the cytoplasm of cells infected with one of the variants of PARA and with nuclear T antigen in cells transformed either by SV40 or by nuclear variants of PARA.

The stability of the SV40 T antigen in the cytoplasm or nucleus was determined by isolating single cells from the *in vitro* transformed 2cT-1 cell line and growing these isolated cells into clonal cell lines. One cell clone was isolated which contained the SV40 T antigen in the cytoplasm and a second cell line contained the T antigen in the nucleus. The localization of the T antigen in each of these cell lines was found to be stable through 60 *in vitro* cell passages. The oncogenic potential of each cell line was also determined as shown in Table 2. The cell clone 2cT-la with cytoplasmic localization of the T antigen was found to induce tumors more rapidly and more frequently than did the cell clone with nuclear localization of the T antigen. Sera from tumor-bearing animals of both cell clones cross-reacted

with both cytoplasmic and nuclear T antigen containing cells. This cross-reaction is direct evidence that the T antigen found in the cytoplasm is closely related if not identical to the nuclear T antigen induced by PARA.

Previous results with PARA variants able to induce the SV40 T antigen in the nucleus have suggested a correlation between ability to induce tumors *in vivo* and the efficiency of *in vitro* cellular transformation (1, 6). The low efficiency of transformation by the cytoplasmic variants of PARA suggests that the oncogenic potential *in vivo* of these variants should be low. Thus far, the injection of the cytoplasmic variants into newborn Syrian hamsters has not yet induced tumor formation. However, the observations that the cells transformed *in vitro* are oncogenic suggest that the number of cells initially transformed is a deciding factor in demonstrating oncogenicity *in vivo* and that the intranuclear localization of the SV40 T antigen is not essential for transformation and oncogenicity following exposure of hamster cells to PARA.

ACKNOWLEDGMENTS

The research upon which this publication is based was supported in part by Grants No. CA 11647 and CA 4600 and Contract No. NIH 70-2024 from the National Institutes of Health, Department of Health, Education, and Welfare.

REFERENCES

1. DUFF, R., and RAPP, F. *J. Virol.* **5**, 568–577 (1970).
2. BUTEL, J. S., GUENTZEL, M. J., and RAPP, F. *J. Virol.* **4**, 632–641 (1969).

3. HARE, J. D., *Virology* **40**, 978-988 (1970).
4. TILZ, G. P., DE VAUX SAINT CYR, CH., and GRABAR, P., *Int. J. Cancer* **4**, 641-647 (1969).
5. BLACK, P. H., *Subviral Carcinogenesis, Int. Symp. Tumor Viruses, Nagoya, Japan,* pp. 220-234 (1967).
6. RAPP, F., PAULUZZI, S., and BUTEL, J. S., *J. Virol.* **4**, 626-631 (1969).

SV40 Virus-induced Tumour Specific Transplantation Antigen in Cultured Mouse Cells

by
RICHARD W. SMITH
JOEL MORGANROTH
PETER T. MORA

TUMOUR specific transplantation antigens (TSTA) which are found in animal tumours[1] and some human cancers[2,3] may be important in host defence against malignancy[4]. Especially significant is the finding that in model animal tumour systems, immunization against a TSTA conveys specific protection against tumours containing that TSTA, presumably through the same immunological mechanisms involved in the rejection of organ transplants.

Until now identification and characterization of TSTAs has been complicated by the lack of procedures for solubilization, purification, and suitable assay. Here we describe simple, rapid *in vitro* assay procedures for SV40 virus-induced TSTA and show that such assays can identify a subcellular fraction possessing *in vivo* immunogenicity and also detect TSTA activity in solubilized tumour cell membranes.

Cell lines transformed by the same DNA virus have a common TSTA, by contrast with chemically induced tumours which possess individually distinct antigens, even when induced by the same carcinogen. RNA virus-transformed cells do possess TSTA, but they also release virus, thus complicating the interpretation of findings. We chose the following non-virus-producing tissue culture cell lines derived from highly inbred AL/N[5] and Balb/c[6] mice to avoid the complication of histocompatibility antigen differences and provide uniform material for biological and biochemical studies[5-7]: (1) N–AL/N : a "normal" non-tumorigenic contact inhibited cell line originally derived from AL/N mouse kidney[5]. (2) T–AL/N: N–AL/N cells spontaneously transformed after the twenty-ninth passage in tissue culture[6]. (3) SV–AL/N: cells obtained from N–AL/N by transformation *in vitro* with a strain of SV40 virus[5]; they contain virus-specific T and transplantation antigens, and produce no infectious virus particles. (4) PY–AL/N: cells similarly obtained by transformation using polyoma virus and containing polyoma T antigen (personal communication from Dr K. K. Takemoto). (5) SV–Balb 3T3: a derivative of 3T3 cells from Balb/c mice[6]. (6) SV–3T3: SV40 transformed 3T3 cells originally derived from non-inbred Swiss mice[9].

SV–AL/N cells do not produce tumours when injected into normal 6 week old Al/N mice but do produce fatal tumours in a high percentage of irradiated (300 rad) mice (Table 1). In the latter group about half of the tumours began to regress 2–3 weeks after irradiation and injection, concurrently with the recovery of immunological competence. This cell line was chosen for further study because of this evidence for the presence of a "strong" TSTA. As also shown in Table 1, PY–AL/N and T–AL/N did not exhibit similar evidence for strong TSTA.

Groups of AL/N mice received 4–12 weekly intramuscular or subcutaneous injections of 10^6 immunizing cells/animal. Similarly, other groups of mice were injected weekly with about 2 mg protein/mouse of a "crude membrane" fraction from SV–AL/N cells. This fraction (designated CM–SV–AL/N) was prepared by a modification[10] of the method originally developed by Davies[11] for the isolation of histocompatibility antigens. The method involves cell disruption by freeze–thawing, elution of membranes by hypotonic salt solution, and high speed centrifugation of these pooled eluted fractions.

Fig. 1 illustrates the abundance of membrane-like structures in the "crude membrane" fraction. The mice were bled 10–14 days after the last injection with the cells or with the "crude membrane". The serum, obtained by centrifugation, was heated to 56° C for 45 min to inactivate complement and stored at −20° C.

Target cells were grown to confluency in suitable culture conditions[8], disaggregated at 37° C for 15–30 min by 0·05 per cent trypsin, and grown overnight in suspension culture. Immediately before use, the cells were washed twice in 0·01 M Tris–HCl buffered saline (pH 7·4) (TBS) and resuspended at a concentration of 10^6/ml. in TBS. Rabbit serum, as a source of complement (Microbiological Associates), was centrifuged for 15 min at $20,000g$ to remove debris and was skimmed while cold to remove a floating lipid layer found to interfere with phase contrast microscopy.

Cytotoxicity reactions were carried out in the wells of microtest tissue culture plates[12] (Falcon Plastics, Los Angeles), using 1 μl. each of diluted mouse serum, undiluted rabbit complement, TBS, and target cell suspension. Complement without serum and serum without complement were always included among the controls. After brief mixing, a drop of mineral oil was added to prevent evaporation, and the plates were incubated at 37° C for 90 min. One μl. of 0·1 per cent trypan blue was then added, the wells were covered with a microscope coverslip, and the cells were observed in the inverted phase contrast microscope. Dead cells stained dark blue with their surface membranes ballooned or disintegrated. Living cells appeared bright and refractile or became attached to the plastic surface and appeared greyish.

Table 1. TUMORIGENICITY* OF MOUSE CELL LINES

Cell line	Dose†	Normal host	Irradiated host‡
SV–AL/N	10^8	0/5	21/25
	10^7	0/40	62/79
	10^6	0/100	8/10
	10^5	0/5	0/5
	10^4	0/5	0/5
	10^3	0/5	0/5
	10^2	0/5	0/5
T–AL/N	10^7	8/8	—
	10^6	10/10	—
	10^5	30/40	5/5
	10^4	3/5	5/5
	10^3	0/5	5/5
PY–AL/N	10^7	10/10	9/13
	10^6	5/5	3/5
	10^5	4/5	—
	10^4	3/5	—

Animals were observed for three months, or until death. Tumours induced by T-AL/N or PY-AL/N cells were observable in 2–3 weeks, did not regress and led to death in 4–6 weeks. Those induced by SV-AL/N cells in irradiated hosts showed about a 50 per cent incidence of complete tumour regression.

* Greater than 0·5 cm nodule at the site of injection.

† Cells/animal injected intramuscularly or subcutaneously.

‡ 300 rad, 16–24 h before subcutaneous or intramuscular injection.

Undiluted positive serum in the presence of complement always gave 95 to 100 per cent target cell death. Serial two-fold dilutions of each serum continued to show 95 to 100 per cent death until a critical dilution at which it fell sharply over the next two or three dilutions. Table 2 shows such a titration. Complement alone and serum alone gave control values ranging between 5 and 20 per cent dead cells. Titres increased with the number of injections received by each group of animals, but each titre was reproducible when the same batch of pooled serum was retested against the same target cell line. Cytotoxic serum was inactive against cells freshly treated with 0·05 per cent trypsin, necessitating growth overnight in suspension culture, possibly to permit regeneration of cell surface constituents.

Specificity Studies

Sera from immunized animals were incubated with various target cells (Table 3). Serum from animals injected with SV-AL/N cells gave cytotoxic reactions with SV40 transformed cells but not with normal, spon-

46

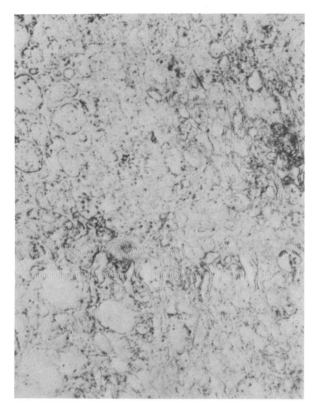

Fig. 1. Electron micrograph of a representative area of a "crude membrane" pellet prepared from SV–AL/N cells. Membrane-like structures and ribosomes abound. Glutaraldehyde–osmium tetroxide fixation, embedding in 'Epon'. Section stained with uranyl acetate and lead citrate. Magnification, ×c. 31,430.

taneously transformed, or polyoma transformed cells of the parent N–AL/N line. The cytotoxic reaction also occurred with SV40 virus-transformed cell lines from Swiss and Balb/c mice (SV–3T3 and SV–BALB/3T3). The "crude membrane" extract from SV–AL/N cells (CM–SV–AL/N) produced antiserum which was likewise specifically cytotoxic. Antisera produced by injection of non-transformed N–AL/N cells were not cytotoxic against any tested cell lines.

To interact with antibody, TSTA, like histocompatibility antigens, must be present on the cell surface. Quantitative antibody absorptions were carried out using whole living cells to determine the magnitude of the difference between virus-transformed cells and control cells in their ability to absorb out cytotoxic antibody (Fig. 2). All three SV40 transformed cell lines tested did absorb out the cytotoxic activity. The control line showed insignificant absorption even at high cell doses. The most potent absorbing cell was the SV–AL/N cell,

Table 2. EFFECT OF ANTISERUM DILUTION ON KILL OF SV-AL/N CELLS

Serum dilution	Per cent dead cells
1	> 95
1/5	> 95
1/10	> 95
1/20	95
1/40	80
1/80	35
1/160	15
Complement, no serum	10
Undiluted serum, no complement	10

Each value represents the mean of four to six determinations.

Table 3. SERUM CYTOTOXICITY TITRES WHICH GAVE GREATER THAN 50 PER CENT CELL DEATH

Antiserum induced by			Target cells			
	SV-AL/N	SV-3T3	SV-Balb/ 3T3	N-AL/N	T-AL/N	PY-AL/N
SV-AL/N	Pos. 1/40	Pos. 1/40	Pos. 1/20	Neg.	Neg.	Neg.
CM-SV- AL/N	Pos. 1/4*	Pos. 1/2	Pos. 1/2	Neg.	Neg.	—
N-AL/N	Neg.	—	—	Neg.	Neg.	—
T-AL/N	Neg.	Neg.	Neg.	Neg.	Neg.	—

Each titre represents mean values using pooled serum from 3-5 groups of 5-10 mice each. All assays were run at least in triplicate.

* An antiserum produced subsequently was active at 1/13 dilution.

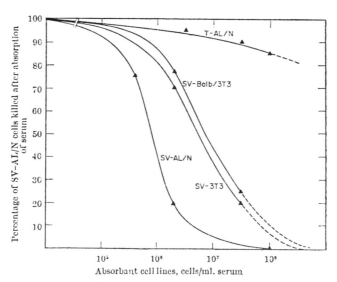

Fig. 2. Cytotoxicity absorption curves. Cytotoxic activity of serum against SV-AL/N cells after absorption with the indicated amounts of living cells from the various cell lines. Serum was diluted so that 95-100 per cent of test cells were killed and any further dilution would result in a sharp decrease in death (Table 2). The diluted serum was incubated with the indicated number of washed, living "absorbant" SV-AL/N, SV-3T3, SV-Balb/3T3, or T-AL/N cells for 60 min at 20° C. with frequent agitation. The cells were removed by centrifugation and the serum was re-tested for residual cytotoxicity against SV-AL/N cells. The volumes were carefully controlled to prevent dilution or concentration.

which has a somewhat larger average size than the SV–Balb/3T3 or SV–3T3 cells. These results confirm the specificity demonstrated in Table 3 and suggest that the SV40 specific TSTA is absent or undetectable on the surface of T–AL/N cells.

Cell Mediated Cytotoxicity

Sensitized lymphocytes are thought to be of primary importance in tissue rejection. Spleens were removed from normal non-sensitized AL/N mice, from mice bearing tumours induced by PY–AL/N cells and from mice immunized by SV–AL/N cells. The spleens were minced, suspended in culture medium, passed through a stainless steel mesh with a pore size of 100 μm, washed twice with Eagle's suspension medium, and then resuspended at a concentration of 10^7 spleen cells/ml. The suspension consisted of approximately 95 per cent mononuclear cells,

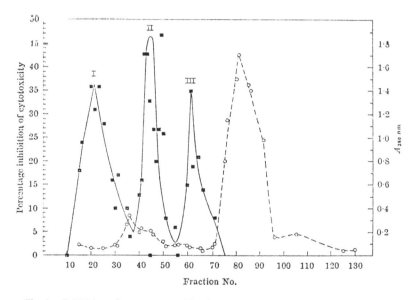

Fig. 3. Inhibition of serum cytotoxicity by fractions of papain-solubilized SV–AL/N "crude membrane" eluted from 'Sephadex G-150'. A column of 1 × 60 cm 'Sephadex G-150' was equilibrated and eluted with 0·01 M Tris–HCl buffered saline (pH 8·6). The solubilized crude membrane fraction was applied to the column in 1 ml. buffer, and 1 ml. fractions were collected at a flow rate of 6 ml./h. The excluded volume, determined by blue dextran, was 18–22 ml. The percentage inhibition of cytotoxicity, representing the mean of 5–10 duplicate determinations on 1 μl. aliquots, is plotted (■ - - - ■). Fractions within the principal 280 nm absorption peak (○ - - - ○) were toxic to the target cells (not shown).

chiefly lymphocytes. Target cells were washed and titred to 10^6/ml. Equal volumes of target and spleen cell suspensions were incubated with gentle shaking at 37° C for 18 h, either in wells of microtest plates (1 μl. of each) or in tightly capped glass tubes (2·5 ml. of each suspension). No complement was added. After incubation overnight in the microtest plates and the addition of trypan blue dye, the percentage of dead tumour cells was determined (Table 4). The much larger tumour cells were easily

Table 4. CELL MEDIATED CYTOTOXICITY (MICROTEST PLATE)

Spleen cells	Target cells		
	SV–AL/N	T–AL/N	PY–AL/N
Immunization:	Per cent killed ± S.D.		
SV–AL/N cells	65 ± 18	11 ± 3	19 ± 6
PY–AL/N cells (tumour bearing)	23 ± 4	8 ± 3	62 ± 6
No immunization	18 ± 9	9 ± 2	15 ± 6
Control (no spleen cells)	10 ± 3	9 ± 3	10

Data compiled from several experiments. An average assay involved six replicate determinations. It was essential to rinse glassware in glass-distilled water and maintain the pH near 7·2 to maintain viability (by dye exclusion test) and cytotoxic activity of the spleen cells.

distinguishable from the spleen cells. SV–AL/N-sensitized spleen cells specifically killed SV-AL/N target cells; the polyoma-sensitized spleen cells specifically killed PY-AL/N target cells. Specific target cell death also occurred using spleen cells both from previously irradiated animals with progressively growing SV–AL/N induced tumours and from non-irradiated animals sensitized to crude membrane from SV–AL/N cells (data not shown). Cytotoxicity was also demonstrated by the reduced ability of target cells to incorporate ^{3}H-thymidine. After overnight incubation of spleen and target cells, thymidine in fresh medium was added to give a final concentration of 2 μCi/ml., and the incubation was continued a further 4 h. After washing and precipitation with trichloroacetic acid, the incorporated radioactivity was determined (Table 5).

The cell mediated cytotoxicity assay (Tables 4 and 5) correlates well with the serum assay (Table 3), but also demonstrates activity which would otherwise be missed. Animals whose serum was positive in the complement-dependent serum cytotoxic assay always yielded spleen cells positive in the cell mediated assay; but animals bearing SV40 or polyoma tumours always had negative serum but positive spleen cells (data not shown).

Table 5. CELL MEDIATED CYTOTOXICITY: UPTAKE OF ^{3}H-THYMIDINE (C.P.M./10⁶ TARGET CELLS)

Sensitized spleen cells	Target cell lines		
	SV–AL/N	PY–AL/N	T–AL/N
SV–AL/N	6,825	4,266	1,463
None	13,181	4,655	1,738

Both serum and cell mediated cytotoxicity assays have been used previously to detect virus induced TSTA (ref. 13). A correlation between *in vitro* sensitivity to cytotoxic antibody and *in vivo* tumour rejection was established in Moloney virus-induced mouse tumour[14]. Likewise, tissue typing by serum cytotoxicity is a good predictor[15] of allogeneic graft rejection in experimental animals[15] and man[16]. We have modified the serum method so that it provides simple, rapid and quantitative assays of TSTA in soluble or insoluble form.

In vivo Protection by Membrane Fragments

Most experiments showing *in vivo* immunization against

50

tumour cells have been done on non-irradiated animals. Takemoto[5] showed, however, that AL/N mice immunized with SV40 virus did not develop tumours after irradiation and challenge inoculation with SV–AL/N cells. As indicated, in our experiments SV–AL/N "crude membrane" induces both serum and spleen cell mediated cytotoxicity —demonstrable *in vitro*. Preliminary data suggest that inoculation with "crude membrane" from SV–AL/N cells also protects syngeneic mice against subsequent tumour cell challenge. AL/N mice were injected twice with 2 mg/animal CM–SV–AL/N. Two other groups were not immunized. Six weeks after the final injection they were bled for cytotoxicity titres, irradiated and challenged with SV–AL/N cells (Table 6). All unimmunized animals developed tumours (see Table 1). No immunized animals developed tumours, indicating protection by immunization with "crude membrane".

Table 6. PROTECTION BY CRUDE MEMBRANE AGAINST SV–AL/N TUMOUR

Immunization	Irradiation	Challenge dose SV–AL/N	Tumours
—	300 rad	1×10^6	5/5
—	300 rad	$1\cdot5 \times 10^6$	4/4
CM–SV–AL/N	300 rad	$5 \times 10^{6*}$	0/5

* At the time of challenge, the serum cytotoxic titre was 1/16.

Unsuccessful attempts by others to immunize hamsters against SV40 TSTA using disrupted cells and microsomal fractions suggested that SV40 TSTA was labile[17]. Our work demonstrates that in mouse cell membranes the antigen is indeed stable and immunogenic.

Subcellular Localization of TSTA

Cells of T–AL/N and SV–AL/N lines were prepared by trypsinization and overnight growth in suspension culture. They were washed in TBS. resuspended in cold 0·25 M sucrose–TBS containing 0·001 M Mg^{2+}, disrupted by nitrogen decompression[18]. from 800 lb/inch², and fractionated by methods similar to those of Wallach and Kamat[19]. Nuclei and cellular debris were sedimented by centrifugation at 600*g* for 5 min. The resulting supernatant, adjusted to 0·002 M with EDTA and centrifuged at 20,000*g* for 10 min, yielded a crude mitochondrial fraction. The supernatant from this fraction was then adjusted to 0·004 M Mg^{2+} and centrifuged at 85,000*g* for 90 min to yield a microsomal pellet and a high speed supernatant.

Subcellular fractions were assayed for their ability specifically to inhibit cytotoxicity. Cytotoxic serum concentration was adjusted to give about 80 per cent cell death in the absence of the inhibitor. One µl. of suitably diluted subcellular fraction, mouse serum, rabbit complement and target cell suspension was incubated as above. The microsomal and mitochondrial fractions of SV–AL/N cells were rich in inhibitory activity compared with the SV–AL/N nuclear and supernatant fractions (Table 7, expt. 1). Microsomal and mitochondrial fractions from T–AL/N cells were not inhibitory (Table 7, exp. 2). Other SV40 induced neoantigens present in the nucleus

51

(T antigen) and on the cell surface (S antigen) have been shown to be unrelated to *in vivo* tumour transplant rejection[20,21], and the recently reported cytoplasmic antigens are also thought to be different from TSTA[22,23]. We have shown that SV40 TSTA is present on the cell surface (Fig. 2) and in membrane-rich subcellular fractions, but is not present in nuclear or soluble cytoplasmic fractions assayed at similar protein concentration.

Solubilization and Partial Fractionation

Solubilization of other TSTAs has been reported[24,25]. Crude membranes were prepared from T-AL/N and from SV-AL/N cells by freeze-thawing and hypotonic salt elution. They were then reacted with papain in conditions known to solubilize histocompatibility antigens[19]. The SV-AL/N particulate crude membrane and the solubilized crude membrane showed specific antigenic activity when assayed by cytotoxicity-inhibition (Table 8). Equivalent fractions from T-AL/N cells were non-inhibitory (data not shown).

The solubilized crude membrane from SV-AL/N cells was passed through a column of 'Sephadex G-150' (Fig. 3). Cytotoxic inhibitory fractions were clearly separated from the principal absorption peak at 280 nm. High-activity material was present in peak I (excluded volume) and in peaks II and III (included volume). The protein concentration in peak II was 123 µg/ml.

Table 7. INHIBITION OF CYTOTOXICITY BY SUBCELLULAR FRACTIONS OF SV-AL/N AND T-AL/N CELLS

Inhibitor fraction	Protein (µg/ml.)	Per cent cell death ± s.d.	Per cent inhibition of cytotoxicity
Expt. 1			
No inhibitor	—	89 ± 4	0
No serum	—	7 ± 3	
No complement	—	3 ± 2	
SV-AL/N nuclear	120	86 ± 4	4
Mitochondrial	165	48 ± 8	48
Microsomal	125	48 ± 12	48
Supernatant	105	84 ± 6	6
Expt. 2			
No inhibitor	—	78	0
No serum	—	28	
No complement	—	28	
SV-AL/N mitochondrial	165	61	36
T-AL/N mitochondrial	665	81	0
T-AL/N mitochondrial	133	80	0
SV-AL/N microsomal	125	50	56
T-AL/N microsomal	400	80	0
T-AL/N microsomal	80	75	6

Subcellular particle fractions were suspended in TBS, assayed for protein by the Lowry method, then suitably diluted. One µl. aliquots were added to the reaction mixture. Incubation and cell counts were done as in the usual cytotoxicity assay. Inhibition of cytotoxicity was calculated by the following formula:

$$\frac{\text{Per cent dead cells with no inhibitor present} - \text{per cent dead cells with inhibitor}}{\text{Per cent dead cells with no inhibitor present} - \text{per cent dead cells in absence of serum or complement}} \times 100$$

Table 8. INHIBITION OF CYTOTOXICITY BY CRUDE MEMBRANE FROM SV-AL/N CELLS AND BY PAPAIN-SOLUBILIZED CRUDE MEMBRANE

Inhibitor	Protein (μg/ml.)	Per cent inhibition
Crude membrane	6,000	100
	3,000	96
	600	15
Solubilized crude membrane (containing papain and iodoacetate)	1,800	60
	900	40
	180	27
Papain and iodoacetate	—	0

To our knowledge this is the first successful solubilization and fractionation of virus-induced TSTA. Further purification will permit biochemical analyses similar to those currently being undertaken with $H2$ and $HL-A$ histocompatibility antigens. Such analyses may also provide a new tool for the study of virus-induced genotypic changes in cells transformed by mutants of DNA viruses. Although *in vitro* assays may not reflect fully the complex *in vivo* situation, their usefulness has been well demonstrated in studies of ordinary transplant antigens.

We have developed simple, rapid *in vitro* assays for SV40 virus-induced TSTA using syngeneic mice and cell lines. The particulate antigen detected by these methods is stable, is present in highest concentration in membrane-rich subcellular fractions, and is immunogenic, eliciting cytotoxic antibody and spleen cells and protecting against tumour cell challenge. Solubilized antigen, detected by cytotoxicity-inhibition, is now being studied for *in vivo* activity. Hopefully, this immunological approach can be applied to RNA virus-induced animal tumours and to human malignancies[2,3] where it may yield clues to their aetiology[26] and ultimately lead to methods for immunoprophylaxis or immunotherapy.

We thank Drs John Wunderlich, John Fahey, Dean Mann and Ronald Herberman for advice. Drs Kenneth Takemoto and George Todaro for cell lines, and Miss Leslie Danoff, Mrs Vivian McFarland, Mr Lorenzo Waters and Mrs Mattie Owens for technical assistance.

[1] Smith, R. T., *New Engl. J. Med.*, 278, 1207 (1968).
[2] Hellström, I., Hellström, K. E., Pierce, G. E., and Yang, J. P. S., *Nature*, 220, 1352 (1968).
[3] Morton, D. L., and Mälmgren, R. A., *Science*, 162, 1279 (1968).
[4] Klein, G., *Fed. Proc.*, 28, 1739 (1969).
[5] Takemoto, K. K., Ting, R. C. Y., Ozer, H. L., and Fabish, P., *J. Nat. Cancer Inst.*, 41, 1401 (1968).
[6] Aaronson, S. A., and Todaro, G. J., *Science*, 162, 1024 (1968).
[7] Kit, S., Kurimura, T., and Dubbs, D. R., *Int. J. Cancer*, 4, 384 (1969).
[8] Mora, P. T., Brady, R. O., Bradley, R. M., and McFarland, V. W., *Proc. US Nat. Acad. Sci.*, 63, 1290 (1969).
[9] Todaro, G. J., and Green, H., *J. Cell. Biol.*, 17, 299 (1963).
[10] Mann, D. L., Rogentine, G. N., Fahey, J. L., and Nathenson, S. G., *J. Immunol.*, 103, 282 (1969).
[11] Davies, D. A. L., *Immunology*, 11, 115 (1966).
[12] Terasaki, P. I., and McClelland, J. D., *Nature*, 204, 998 (1964).
[13] Hellström, I., and Sjögren, H. O., *J. Exp. Med.*, 125, 1105 (1967).
[14] Klein, G., Klein, E., and Haughton, G., *J. Nat. Cancer Inst.*, 36, 607 (1966).
[15] Snell, G. D., and Stimpfling, J. H., in *The Biology of the Laboratory Mouse* (McGraw-Hill, New York, 1966).
[16] Terasaki, P. I., Vrdevoe, D. L., and Mickey, M. R., *Transplantation Supplement*, 1967.

[17] Panteleakis, P. N., Larson, V. M., Glenn, E. S., and Hilleman, M. R., *Proc. Soc. Exp. Biol. Med.*, **129**, 50 (1968).

[18] Hunter, M. J., and Commerford, S. L., *Biochim. Biophys. Acta*, **47**, 580 (1961).

[19] Wallach, D. F. H., and Kamat, V. B., *Methods in Enzymology*, **8**, 16 (1966).

[20] Black, P. H., Rowe, W. P., Turner, H. C., and Huebner, R. J., *Proc. US Nat. Acad. Sci.*, **50**, 1148 (1963).

[21] Tevethia, S. S., Diamandopoulos, G. T., Rapp, F., and Enders, J. *Immunol.*, **101**, 1192 (1968).

[22] Saint Cyr, Ch. de V., Herbert, A., Sobczak, E., Wicker, R., and Grabar, P., *Intern. J. Cancer*, **4**, 616 (1969).

[23] Tilz, G. P., Saint Cyr, Ch. de V., and Grabar, P., *Intern. J. Cancer*, **4**, 641 (1969).

[24] Oettgen, H. F., Old, L. J., McLean, E. P., and Carewell, E. A., *Nature*, **220**, 295 (1968).

[25] Davies, D. A. L., Boyse, E. A., Old, L. J., and Stockert, E., *J. Exp. Med.*, **125**, 549 (1967).

[26] Huebner, R. J., and Todaro, G. J., *Proc. US Nat. Acad. Sci.* (in the press).

Induction of Simian Virus 40 Antigen in BSC₁ Transformed Cells

MIRIAM MARGALITH, EVA MARGALITH, TAMAR NASIALSKI, AND N. GOLDBLUM

Infectious simian virus 40 (SV40) can be recovered from SV40 transformed cells by cocultivation or fusion with susceptible monkey kidney cells. Rescue of the virus is facilitated by the use of ultraviolet inactivated Sendai virus for fusion (3, 4, 6, 11, 12, 13, 14, 16, 19, 21).

The transformation of BSC_1 cells by SV40 virus was previously reported by Margalith et al. (16). This report describes the induction of SV40 viral antigen, but not infectious virus, in cloned virus-free BSC_1 transformed cells. However, infectious virus can be recovered by other methods such as cell fusion or mitomycin C, indicating the presence of complete viral genomes.

MATERIALS AND METHODS

Cells, media, and chemicals. The SV40 transformed BSC_1 cloned cells (16) were grown in Eagle's basal medium containing four times the concentration of amino acids and vitamins (Eagle's modified) supplemented with 10% calf serum.

The monkey kidney BSC_1 cell line was obtained from Microbiological Associates, Bethésda, Md., and grown in Eagle's modified medium supplemented with 10% calf serum.

The rabbit kidney cell line, MA-111, was obtained from Microbiological Associates, Bethesda, Mu. It was adapted in our laboratory to growth in Eagle's modified medium supplemented with 10% calf serum. According to a personal communication from Klaus Schell, Microbiological Associates, this cell line is as sensitive to the cytolytic effect of SV40 virus as the BSC_1 cell line. We were able to confirm these findings in our laboratory. These findings were also reported by Schell and Maryak (18a).

Mitomycin C was obtained from Kyowa Hakko Kogyo Co. Ltd., Tokyo, Japan, and cytosine arabinoside from Sigma Chemical Co., St. Louis, Mo.

Immunofluorescent technique. This was done on cells grown in Leighton tubes on cover slips. According to the experiment, cover slips were withdrawn, washed three times with Hanks solution, washed twice with acetone, and fixed with acetone for 3 min. They were then dried and stored at -70 C. For the detection of the viral antigen, the cover slips were stained for 30 min at 37 C with 1:4 dilution of the antiviral SV40 serum. The antiserum was coupled with fluorescein isothiocyanate as described by Ravid et al. (18). The gamma globulin fraction was separated on a diethyl-aminoethyl cellulose column by using phosphate buffer (0.01 M, pH 7.2) supplemented with 0.15 M NaCl. Monkey antiviral SV40 serum was kindly supplied by J. L. Melnick, College of Medicine, Baylor University, Houston, Tex.

Infectivity titrations. These were made on BSC_1 monolayers in tubes or in 60-mm petri dishes (Falcon Plastic, Div. of B-D Laboratories Inc., Los Angeles, Calif.). The BSC_1 monolayers were washed with Hanks solution and inoculated with 0.5 ml of the appropriate virus dilution. The inoculum was adsorbed for 3 hr at 37 C. The tube monolayers were observed during 3 weeks for the characteristic cytopathic effect. The monolayers in the petri dishes were overlaid as reported previously (16). For the plaque assay the monolayers were stained 3 weeks after inoculation. Plaques were visible 10 to 24 hr after staining.

Cell-fusion technique. The method used was a modified version of that described by Harris et al. (9) and by Watkins and Dulbecco (21). Cells were diluted in Hanks solution at 4 C. To 1.5 ml of a cell mixture composed of 3×10^6 transformed BSC_1 cells and 3×10^5 rabbit kidney cells, 1.5 ml of ultraviolet-inactivated Sendai virus, containing 400 hemagglutinating (HA) units, was added. The cell mixture was kept in an ice bath for 15 min and then placed in a 37 C water bath and shaken for an additional 20 min. The cells were then further processed as follows: (i) they were seeded on BSC_1 monolayers, adsorbed 2 hr, and overlaid with an agar overlay as described (assay for infectious centers), or (ii) the cell mixture was suspended in 10 ml of Eagle's modified medium, containing 10% calf serum, and the cells were seeded in Falcon petri dishes; the medium was changed after 24 hr, and the monolayers which grew out in the plates were harvested 1 to 3 weeks later and assayed for infectious virus on BSC₁ cells.

Preparation of ultraviolet-inactivated Sendai virus. Ten-day-old chick embryos were inoculated with 10⁵ Sendai virus (received from A. Kohn, Israel Institute for Biological Research, Nes Ziona, Israel) by the allantoic route. After incubation at 37 C for 48 hr and refrigeration overnight, the allantoic fluids were harvested. The fluids were centrifuged at $1,000 \times g$ for 15 min and then at $30,000 \times g$ for 1 hr. The pellet was resuspended in Hanks solution at 0.5 the original volume. Inactivation was carried out by exposure of 3 ml of the virus in 60-mm petri dishes for 3 min to ultraviolet radiation at a dose of 1,550 ergs per cm² per sec.

RESULTS

Induction of SV40 viral antigen. BSC₁-transformed cells were grown on cover slips in Leighton tubes. On the fourth day the growth medium was changed to Eagle's modified medium supplemented with 2% calf serum, and the tubes were placed in a 45 C water bath for various periods of time ranging from 10 to 60 min. After heating, the cells were incubated at 34 C for 96 hr, and samples were withdrawn every 24 hr for immunofluorescent staining and infectivity tests. In each of six experiments, approximately 10,000 cells were counted in each duplicate preparation and the percentage of cells synthesizing viral antigen was determined. In preliminary experiments a direct relationship was found between the percentage of cells synthesizing viral antigen and the time of heating to 45 C, up to 1 hr. A 30-min interval was chosen for the majority of the experiments, as this treatment caused least cell destruction and optimum induction. Figure 1 shows the appearance of SV40 viral antigen in BSC₁ transformed cells after heating at 45 C for 30 min as a function of the time of incubation. The highest percentage of cells exhibiting viral antigen was found after 3 days. For infectivity tests, samples of 10⁶ and 10⁵ cells with the medium were frozen and thawed twice, sonically treated, and tested for infectious virus by plating on BSC₁ monolayers in petri dishes and in tubes. No infectious virus was detected from numerous samples of the induced cells tested, although all exhibited viral antigen.

We were able to induce a larger number of cells to synthesize viral antigen after heating at 45 C for 30 min by withdrawing arginine from the medium. In these experiments transformed BSC₁ cell monolayers were washed twice with Hanks solution,

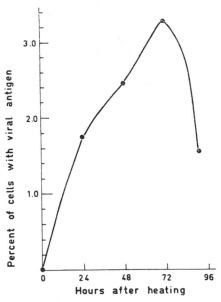

Fig. 1. *Induction of simian virus 40 (SV40) viral antigen by heating to 45 C for 30 min. SV40-transformed BSC₁ cells grown on cover slips in Leighton tubes were subjected to heating at 45 C for 30 min. After this treatment they were incubated at 34 C, samples were withdrawn every 24 hr for immunofluorescent staining, and the percentage of cells synthesizing viral antigen was determined.*

and Eagle's medium, depleted of arginine and supplemented with 2% dialyzed calf serum, was added. The monolayers were heated to 45 C for 30 min and then incubated at 34 C. Duplicate samples for immunofluorescent staining and for infectivity titrations were withdrawn every 24 hr for 4 days. In the monolayers with arginine-depleted medium, the percentage of cells exhibiting viral antigen was two to three times higher than in the monolayers kept with regular medium. In addition, the percentage of cells exhibiting viral antigen was the highest 48 hr after heating. No infectious virus was recovered from these cells in any of the samples tested.

Effect of cytosine arabinoside (ara-C) on the induction of SV40 viral antigen. We used ara-C to study the effect of inhibition of DNA synthesis on the induction of viral antigen by heat. BSC₁ transformed cell monolayers in Leighton tubes were heated to 45 C for 30 min, 10 μg/ml of ara-C was added, and the tubes were incubated at 34 C. Samples were removed at 48 and 72 hr later for immunofluorescence. Ara-C inhibited completely the induction of SV40 viral antigen, indicating that deoxyribonucleic acid (DNA) synthesis is necessary for the induction process (Table 1).

Reactivation of infectious virus from BSC₁-transformed cells. Fusion experiments with susceptible BSC₁ cells did not cause the reactivation of SV40 virus. Negative results in fusion experiments with monkey kidney cells were also reported by F. Rapp, Baylor University, College of Medicine, Houston, Tex. (*personal communication*). However, infectious SV40 was rescued by fusing BSC₁ transformed cells with rabbit kidney cells, the MA111 cell line. Infectious SV40 virus was rescued by each of the two methods used: (i) growing the cells after fusion into monolayers and seeding samples of cells and medium at weekly intervals on BSC₁ indicator cells, or (ii) by plating the cells after fusion on BSC₁ monolayers and determining the number of infectious centers. The amount of virus recovered was small in all experiments. It was highest at 3 weeks after fusion, amounting to 1.5×10^2 plaque-forming units (PFU) per 10^6 BSC₁ transformed cells. The infectious center assay indicated that 1 out of 25,000 cells yielded infectious SV40 virus.

Infectious SV40 could also be recovered from the BSC₁ transformed cells by treatments with mitomycin C (5, 8; M. Fogel and L. Sacho, Virology, *in press*). The concentrations of mitomycin C used were 2.5, 5, 7.5, and 10 µg/ml. Grown out monolayers were treated with mitomycin C for 24 hr. The mitomycin was then removed, and fresh Eagle's modified medium with 2% calf serum was added. The monolayers were incubated at 34 C, and samples were withdrawn after 72 and 96 hr and assayed for infectivity on BSC₁ monolayers. Infectious virus was rescued from transformed cells treated with 7.5 and 10 µg of mitomycin C, but not from cells treated with lower concentrations. Ca. 40 PFU of infectious virus were recovered from a tube culture, which contained 2×10^5 transformed cells.

DISCUSSION

It has been shown in recent years that virus transformed cells contain a number of copies of the viral genome and that fully infectious virus can be rescued from such cells (3, 4, 6, 11–14, 16, 19, 21). The mechanism of reactivation of infectious virus is as obscure as the oncogenesis process itself.

This report which deals with the mechanisms of induction may constitute a contribution to the understanding of the processes involved in viral oncogenesis. We have shown that heating of SV40-transformed BSC₁ cells to 45 C induces the synthesis of viral antigen, without concomitant production of infectious virus. The fact that heat treatment causes induction of viral antigen only might have been explained by the presence of a defective viral genome in SV40 transformed BSC₁ cells. However, the reactivation experiments—both by cell fusion with rabbit kidney cells and by treatment with mitomycin C—indicate that the viral genome is not defective (at least in a fraction of the cells) and that all viral functions can be fully expressed.

The induction of viral antigen may be explained in a number of ways. (i) Heat treatment induces a part of the repressed viral genome only (partial derepression). This would indicate that the viral genome in the transformed cells is under a complex repression system and that induction of viral antigen is caused by heat inactivation of one of the heat labile repressors. Examples of heat labile

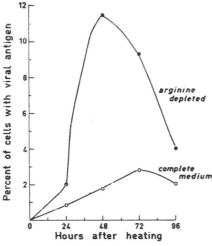

Fig. 2. *Induction of simian virus 40 (SV40) viral antigen by heating to 45 C for 30 min, with and without arginine. For details, see legend to Fig. 1.*

Table 1. *Effect of cytosine arabinoside on the induction of SV40 viral antigen in BSC₁ transformed cells*

Time after heating[a]	Percentage of cells induced	
	With ara-C	Without ara-C
hr		
48	0	2.2
72	0	3.8

[a] At 45 C for 30 min.

repressors have been reported in other systems (10, 15, 17). The synthesis of SV40 viral antigen would thus represent only one event in a series of events involved in the rescue of infectious virus from the transformed cells. (ii) Heating of the transformed cells affects selectively the synthesis of one of the viral coat proteins (1, 2). Since the synthesis of the viral antigens was determined by the immunofluorescence technique, it is possible that this method detects only one of the viral coat proteins and not the others, and (iii) heat treatment induces the synthesis of all viral coat proteins but, for some unexplained reason, viral maturation is blocked in the induced cells and, therefore, no infectious viral progeny is produced.

The molecular events leading to the synthesis of viral antigen in the heat-treated cells are not understood at present and are currently under study. The inhibition of the synthesis of viral antigen by cytosine arabinoside undoubtly indicates the necessity in the induction process of DNA synthesis, viral, cellular, or both. Ara-C was shown to inhibit rescue of infectious virus from SV40-transformed cells (11) and may have a similar effect in our system. The effect of arginine depletion on the induction of the viral antigen also needs further clarification. In this study, depletion in arginine resulted in the increase of viral protein synthesis after heat treatment. In an earlier study, we have reported that arginine is essential for the synthesis of viral coat protein during the replication of SV40 virus (7). These seem to be somewhat contradictory findings and require further investigation.

LITERATURE CITED

1. Anderer, F. A., H. D. Schlumberger, M. A. Koch, H. Frank, and H. J. Eggers. 1967. Structure of simian virus 40. II. Symmetry and components of the virus particle. Virology 32:511–523.
2. Anderer, F. A., M. A. Koch, and H. D. Schlumberger. 1968. Structure of simian virus 40. III. Alkaline degradation of the virus particle. Virology 34:452–458.
3. Dubbs, D. R., and S. Kit. 1968. Isolation of defective lysogens from simian virus 40-transformed mouse kidney cultures. J. Virol. 2:1272–1282.
4. Dubbs, D. R., and S. Kit. 1969. Heterokaryon formation of simian virus 40-transformed cells in the presence of ultraviolet-irradiated Sendai virus. J. Virol. 3:536–538.
5. Gerber, P. 1964. Virogenic hamster tumor cells. Induction of virus synthesis. Science 145:833.
6. Gerber, P. 1966. Studies on the transfer of subviral infectivity from SV40-induced hamster tumor cells to indicator cells. Virology 28:501–509.
7. Goldblum, N., Z. Ravid, and Y. Becker. 1968. Effect of withdrawal of arginine and other amino acids on the synthesis of tumour and viral antigens of SV40 virus. J. Gen. Virol. 31:143–146.
8. Haas, M., and H. Yoshikawa. 1969. Defective bacteriophage PBSH in Bacillus subtilis. I. Induction, purification, and physical properties of the bacteriophage and its deoxyribonucleic acid. J. Virol. 3:233–247.
9. Harris, H., J. F. Watkins, G. E. Ford, and G. I. Schoefli. 1966. Artificial heterokaryons of animal cells from different species. J. Cell Sci. 1:1–30.
10. Horiuchu, T., and A. Novick. 1961. A thermolabile repression system. Cold Spring Harbor Symp. Quant. Biol. 26:247–248.
11. Kit, S., T. Kurimura, M. L. Salvi, and D. R. Dubbs. 1968. Activation of infectious SV40 DNA synthesis in transformed cells. Proc. Nat. Acad. Sci. U.S.A. 60:1239–1246.
12. Kit, S., T. Kurimura, R. A. C. Torres, and D. R. Dubbs. 1969. Simian virus 40 deoxyribonucleic acid replication. I. Effect of cycloheximide on the replication of SV40 DNA in monkey kidney cells and in heterokaryons of SV40-transformed and susceptible cells. J. Virol. 3:25–32.
13. Knowles, B. B., F. C. Jenzen, L. Steplewski, and H. Koprowski. 1968. Rescue of SV40 virus after fusion between different SV40 transformed cells. Proc. Nat. Acad. Sci. U.S.A. 61:42–45.
14. Koprowski, H., F. C. Jensen, and Z. Steplewski. 1967. Activation of production of infectious tumor virus SV40 in heterokaryons cultures. Proc. Nat. Acad. Sci. U.S.A. 58: 127–133.
15. Lieb ,M. 1966. Studies of heat-inducible lambda bacteriophage. I. Order of genetic sites and properties of mutant prophages. J. Mol. Biol. 16:149–163.
16. Margalith, M., R. Volk-Fuchs, and N. Goldblum. 1969. Transformation of BSC₁ cells following chronic infection with SV40. J. Gen. Virol. 5:321–327.
17. Novick, A., E. S. Lennox, and F. Jacob. 1963. Relationship between rate of enzyme synthesis and repressor level. Cold Spring Harbor Symp. Quant. Biol. 28:397–401.
18. Ravid, Z., M. Margalith, and N. Goldblum. 1968. Rapid titration of high concentrations of SV40 virus by immunofluorescence. Isreal J. Med. Sci. 4:945–948.
18a. Schell, K., and J. Maryak. 1967. SV40 virus growth and cytopathogenicity in a serial rabbit kidney cell line. Proc. Soc. Exp. Biol. Med. 124:1099–1102.
19. Takemoto, K. K., G. J. Todaro, and S. K. Habel. 1968. Rescue of SV40 virus with genetic markers of original inducing virus from SV40 transformed cells. Virology 35:1–8.
20. Tal, H. T., and L. R. O'Brien. 1969. Multiplicity of viral genomes in an SV40 transformed hamster cell line. Virology 38:698–701.
22. Watkins, J. F., and R. Dulbecco. 1967. Production of SV40 virus in heterokaryons of transformed and susceptible cells. Proc. Nat. Acad. Sci. U.S.A. 58:1396–1403.

Antigenic Study of Unfertilized Mouse Eggs:
Cross Reactivity with SV40-Induced Antigens*

Wanda Baranska, Pavel Koldovsky, and Hilary Koprowski

The antigenicity of mammalian ova has been studied primarily in immunologic reactions against fertilized eggs. The results of these investigations indicate that mouse embryos apparently can divide unhampered when implanted in nonimmunized allogeneic,[1,2] single skin-graft immunized, or even xenogeneic hosts,[3,4] and that only hyperimmunization of the recipient animals may prevent their growth.[5,6]

Blastocysts grown *in vitro* without zona pellucida were found to be immunosensitive to the action of cells and serum obtained from an immunized animal,[7,8] but the presence of the zona pellucida seemed to decrease their immunosensitivity to immune serum[7,8] without affecting their susceptibility to the effect of immune cells.[7]

In addition to evidence for the presence of adult alloantigens, the existence of embryo-specific antigens has been postulated because repeated transfer of allogeneic blastocysts into male mice caused inhibition of development of subsequently implanted allogeneic and syngeneic blastocysts.[9]

In contrast to the above studies, we have investigated in this paper unfertilized mouse eggs with heteroimmune sera, hoping to gain information about antigenic properties of a mammalian ovum at the earliest stage of development.

Materials and Methods. **Egg cells:** Unfertilized eggs were obtained either from 8- to 10-week-old C57BL/6 or BALB-C virgin mice according to the technique described elsewhere.[10] The cumulus oöphorus was removed by treatment with hyaluronidase.[11]

For immunization, the cells were washed twice in Brinster's medium (BMOC₂),[12] resuspended in 0.25 ml of BMOC₂, and disrupted by squeezing back and forth through a syringe. The contents of approximately 100 eggs were then mixed with 0.25 ml of complete Freund's adjuvant (Difco, catalog no. 0638-59).

For cytotoxicity tests, additional eggs were obtained from 5-week-old Wistar virgin rats treated with hormones for superovulation.[13] After removal of the cumulus oöphorus, the zona pellucida was removed from mouse and rat eggs by treatment with a 0.25%

59

solution of pronase.[14]   The cells were then washed three times in $BMOC_2$ and maintained in this medium at room temperature until exposed to serum.

Somatic cells: MC57G and MBG are permanent tissue culture cell lines originating from methylcholanthrene-induced tumors in adult C57BL/6 (MC57G) and CBA (MBG) mice.   PF-1 is a cell line originating from SV40-transformed C57BL/6 embryonic tissue.[15]   The 3T3 is a line originating from normal Swiss mouse embryonic tissue, and the 3T3-SV is the same cell line transformed by SV40.[16]   Lymph-node cells were obtained from normal adult C57BL/6 mice.

Cytotoxicity test: Seven to 21 mouse eggs, without the zona pellucida (see above), were placed in 0.05 ml of $BMOC_2$, at pH 7.4, in a small Petri dish and exposed to 0.05 ml of the respective dilutions of serum.   The mixture was incubated at 37°C in a CO_2 atmosphere, and the results were recorded after an incubation time of 30 min.   When inactivated serum was used in the test, groups of egg cells were first exposed to the inactivated serum and, after 10 min incubation, a drop of fresh guinea pig complement was added to the mixture.   As a control, serum obtained from guinea pigs injected only with complete Freund's adjuvant was used.

The cytotoxicity test performed on the somatic cells has been described by Bodmer *et al.*[17]; fluorescein acetate was used to stain the viable cells.

Colony inhibition test: The technique described by Hellström and Sjögren[18] was used, with the exception that fresh guinea pig serum was used as a source of complement instead of rabbit serum.

Membrane immunofluorescence of the somatic cells: The method described by Möller[19] was followed.   The anti-mouse egg serum and the control guinea pig serum were heat inactivated, and the rabbit anti-guinea pig gammaglobulin, labeled with fluorescein (Hyland Laboratories, Los Angeles, Calif.), was absorbed with an excess of MC57G cells before use in the immunofluorescence test.

Sera: An adult female guinea pig weighing 300 g received intradermally seven injections of unfertilized C57BL/6 eggs in complete Freund's adjuvant (see above) twice weekly.   A total of 1239 eggs was injected during a $3\frac{1}{2}$-week period.   Blood was obtained by heart puncture one day after the last injection, and the separated serum was stored at -25°C.

The control animal received the same number of injections consisting of complete Freund's adjuvant alone.   Either fresh serum or serum inactivated at 56°C for 30 min was used.   Fresh guinea pig serum was used as the source of complement.   Absorption of anti-egg guinea pig serum was carried out by mixing 0.3 ml of 1:10 diluted immune serum with packed cells: 10^7 of PF-1 or 3×10^7 of MC57G.   The mixture was kept for 1 hr at room temperature and for another hour at 4°C with occasional shaking of the tubes.

Serum that contained H-2B antibody was prepared in DBA/2 mice by Dr. Joy Palm of this Institute.   During a one-week period, mice were given one subcutaneous and two intraperitoneal injections of a mixture of spleen, thymus, lymph-node, and liver cells from C57BL/6 mice.   The mice were reinjected intraperitoneally 50 days later with the same inoculum and were bled 6 days after the last inoculation.

Results. Reactivity of eggs in cytotoxicity test: Results (Table 1) indicate that serum produced in guinea pigs against C57BL/6 eggs (referred to hereafter as AE serum) was cytotoxic for unfertilized eggs obtained from either BALB-C or C57BL/6 mice. When titrated against C57BL/6 eggs, the end point of the cytotoxic reaction was reached at a dilution of 1:80 of the immune serum. No cytotoxic reaction was observed when rat eggs were exposed to AE serum.

Control guinea pig sera had no effect on either BALB-C or C57BL/6 eggs. The cytotoxic reaction was apparently complement dependent because it was abolished after inactivation of the serum by heat but restored by the addition of fresh guinea pig serum.

TABLE 1. *Effect of guinea pig anti-C57BL/6 egg serum on unfertilized eggs of syngeneic, allogeneic, or xenogeneic origin.*

Origin of eggs	Serum	Undiluted	1:5	1:10	1:20	1:40	1:80
C57BL/6	I		14/14	14/14	8/8	12/17	0/16
	I-inactivated	0/14†	0/14				
	I-inactivated + complement*	6/14	4/14				
	Complement*	1/6					
	C or CA	0/20		0/20			
BALB-C	I		10/10		10/10		
	C	0/7					
Rat	I	0/21					

I = immune serum.
C = prebleeding specimen of serum of guinea pig subsequently immunized with mouse eggs.
CA = serum obtained from guinea pig treated with adjuvant only.
* 1:10 dilution of guinea pig serum.
† Numerator = number of eggs observed; denominator = number of eggs destroyed.

TABLE 2. *Effect of guinea pig anti-C57BL/6 egg serum on somatic mouse cells of syngeneic and allogeneic origin.*

Strain of mice	Cells	Serum	Assays		
			Cytotoxicity	Colony inhibition†	Immuno-fluorescence
C57BL/6	MC57G (MC-induced tumor)	I	46/206*	70	65/91 70/107‡
		CA	31/127	94	11/96
		C			9/118‡
		C			3/123
		C			7/97
	PF-1 (SV40-transformed embryonic cells)	I	65/112 46/113‡	4	57/106
		C	16/100 23/108‡	189	11/83
	Lymph-node cells	I	42/120		
		C	49/111		
Swiss	3T3-SV (SV40-transformed 3T3 cells)	I	50/98		
		C	19/106		
	3T3 ("normal" embryonic cells)	I	25/114		
		CA	26/116		
CBA	MBG (MC-induced tumor)	I	16/140	14	39/102
		C	25/115	12	99/104

For I and CA definitions see footnote to Table 1.
C = prebleeding specimen (footnote to Table 1) or sera from randomly bled normal guinea pigs.
* Numerator = number of cells observed; denominator = number of cells either destroyed in cytotoxicity test or showing membrane fluorescence in the immunofluorescence test.
† Average number of colonies growing out of 300 seeded cells.
‡ Second test with the same serum performed three weeks later.

Effect of AE serum on somatic cells: As shown in Table 2, AE serum was not cytotoxic for MC57G and MBG tumor cells; nor was it cytotoxic for 3T3 cells originating from mouse embryo. No cytotoxicity was observed in the reaction between AE serum and lymph-node cells obtained from normal adult C57BL/6 mice. The results of colony inhibition tests confirmed the lack of cytotoxicity of the serum for MBG cells, whereas the results obtained in the same test with MC57G cells were equivocal.

In contrast, the results of repeated cytotoxicity and colony-inhibition assays with SV40-transformed PF-1 cells of C57BL/6 origin indicate that the AE serum was definitely cytotoxic for these cells. The AE serum was also cytotoxic for the 3T3 cells transformed by SV40 (3T3-SV).

In the immunofluorescence test, a larger proportion of all cells tested (Table 2) showed membrane fluorescence in the presence of AE serum than in the presence of either of the control sera. Figure 1 shows the membrane-type fluorescence observed with MC57G cells. It should be noted that the fluorescent "ring" is not of uniform density around the cell but shows patches of "denser" fluorescent staining at various points on the membrane.

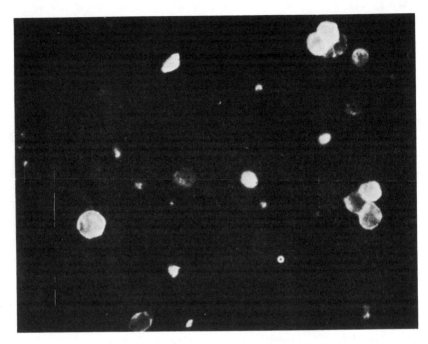

Fig. 1. Ring immunofluorescence of MC57G cells treated with guinea pig anti-C57BL/6 egg serum. Note denser fluorescent-stained patches at various points on the cell membranes. ×400.

Effect of mouse anti-C57BL/6 serum on mouse eggs: Serum produced in DBA/2 mice against C57BL/6 somatic (spleen) cells was cytotoxic (Table 3) for C57BL/6 lymph-node cells but not for C57BL/6 eggs.

Effect of further immunization of guinea pig on reactivity of its serum: In order to investigate the possibility that the exposure of the guinea pig to C57BL/6 egg antigen was insufficient to produce a serum which cross reacted more vigorously with the somatic cells, the animal described above received two more

TABLE 3. *Lack of effect of anti-C57BL/6 serum on mouse eggs of syngeneic origin.*

Cells	Ratio of cells destroyed after exposure to serum dilutions			
	Undiluted	1:2	1:4	1:8
Mouse eggs	0/10	0/20		
Lymph-node cells	83/91	66/74	87/146	47/112

series of injections of C57BL/6 eggs in complete Freund's adjuvant. A serum specimen was obtained one week after the last injection and bioassayed. The results show no difference from those obtained with serum tested after the initial injections of antigen.

Absorption of antibodies from AE serum: As shown in Table 4, the cytotoxic

TABLE 4. *Cytotoxicity test on C57BL/6 eggs with anti-egg serum absorbed with PF-1 and MC57G cells.*

Anti-egg serum diluted 1:10 adsorbed with cells	Ratio of eggs destroyed
PF-1	2/30
MC57G	18/29
None	26/29

reaction of C57BL/6 eggs was virtually eliminated after absorption of AE serum with PF-1 cells. Following absorption with MC57G cells, 18 out of 29 eggs of C57BL/6 were destroyed as compared to 26 out of 29 destroyed after exposure to untreated serum.

Discussion. The results presented in this paper indicate that unfertilized mouse ova, at the one-cell stage, show the presence of an antigen which induces in immunized guinea pigs formation of an antibody cytotoxic not only for eggs of the donor strain but also for eggs obtained from a strain of mice which differs from the donor strain at the H-2 locus. The anti-egg antibody was not cytotoxic for rat eggs and may, therefore, be considered as species-specific. Furthermore, the egg antigen is probably not an H-2 antigen since serum containing H-2B antibody, which destroyed C57BL/6 lymph-node cells, was not cytotoxic for C57BL/6 eggs. This finding seems to confirm the observations of Heyner *et al.*[8] who found no evidence for the presence of H-2 antigens in eight-cell embryos obtained from fertilized mice.

The cross-reactivity of the AE serum with antigens present in the somatic cells of syngeneic and allogeneic strains of mice must be interpreted in the light of the particular test employed. In the cytotoxicity test, the AE serum failed to react with lymph-node cells obtained from the syngeneic adult mice of the C57BL/6 strain or with the 3T3 cells of "normal" embryonic origin. The AE serum was also nonreactive in cytotoxicity and colony-inhibition tests with malignant cells of syngeneic and allogeneic origin obtained from methylcholanthrene-induced tumors. In the immunofluorescence test, positive membrane fluorescence was observed in 70% of MC57G cells, in 50% of PF-1 cells, and in 40% of MBG cells (Table 2). These differences indicate *per se* how less sure one can be in interpreting results of the immunofluorescence test than either cytotoxicity or colony-inhibition tests. The fact, however, that absorption with MC57G cells seemed to decrease somewhat the cytotoxicity of AE serum for C57BL/6 eggs may, perhaps, suggest the presence on the surface of these and other somatic cells of a "weak" antigen cross reacting with AE serum only in an immunofluorescence test. Whether the "patchy" fluorescence pattern reflects distribution of the antigen at different concentrations on the cell membrane is difficult to state at present.

What is, perhaps, most interesting was the cross reactivity of AE serum with the SV40-transformed mouse PF-1 and 3T3-SV cells. In contrast to results obtained with the other somatic cells, including those of "normal" embryonic origin, this reactivity with PF-1 cells was observed in the cytotoxicity and colony-inhibition tests and with 3T3-SV cells in cytotoxicity tests. The cross reactivity between the SV40-transformed cells and mouse eggs was further supported by the virtual elimination of cytotoxicity of AE serum for C57BL/6 eggs after absorption by PF-1 cells.

Parallel suggestive evidence of relationships between transplantation antigens present in polyoma-transformed hamster cells and antigens present in normal embryonic hamster tissue was presented some time ago.[20] Although direct evidence for such a relationship between SV40-transformed cells and their embryonic counterparts is still lacking, one may, perhaps, draw some conclusions from the study of the antigenic makeup of mouse cells treated with proteases and of cells transformed by SV40. Using an agglutinin isolated from wheat germ lipase, Burger[21] observed that whereas mouse and hamster cells transformed by either polyoma or SV40(3T3-SV) are agglutinated without any prior treatment, normal cells of the same origin will only agglutinate after treatment with proteases. In the light of these results, Burger[21] postulates that viral transformation changes the structure of the cell surface sufficiently to unearth receptor sites "masked" in the normal cell. Of even more direct interest to our findings is the observation of Häyry and Defendi[15], that on the surface of hamster cells treated with proteases, there is an antigen which reacts "specifically" with anti-SV40 serum in the mixed hemagglutination test. Thus, the antigen of the PF-1 and 3T3-SV cells, induced by SV40 transformation, may represent nothing more than an antigen already present in the one-cell ovum which is not expressed in adult normal tissue, but which can be derepressed by transformation of the cells with SV40. Whether this antigen is identical with "normal" cell antigen unmasked by treatment with proteases has still to be investigated. It seems clear, however, that this antigen is not detected, in the cytotoxicity and colony inhibition tests, on cells which originate from tumor tissue induced by chemical carcinogens or from normal embryonic tissue, but is detected on cells transformed by one of the oncogenic viruses.

Many studies have reported antigenic cross reactivity between embryonal and malignant tissue.[22-25] In the light of our results, it would be of interest to determine the incidence of the sharing of embryonal antigen, at the earliest stage of development, with malignant cell antigen, regardless of origin or method of transformation. In addition, it would be interesting to study the fate of this antigen in the course of embryonic development in order to determine precisely the time of appearance of the normal "adult" transplantation antigen.

The authors wish to acknowledge the helpful suggestions of Dr. Joy Palm of this Institute and Dr. Niels K. Jerne of the Basel Institute for Immunology, Basel, Switzerland. Dr. E. M. Fenyö, of the Dept. of Tumor Biology, Karolinska Institute, Stockholm, Sweden, kindly supplied the MBG tissue culture line.

* This investigation was supported in part by Public Health Service Research grants S01-FR 05540 from the General Research Support Branch, R01-CA 04534 and P01-CA 10815 from the National Cancer Institute; and funds from The Lalor Foundation.

[1] Kirby, D. R. S., *Nature*, **187**, 707 (1960).
[2] Simmons, R. L., and P. S. Russell, *Ann. N. Y. Acad. Sci.*, **99**, 717 (1962).
[3] Warwick, B. L., and R. O. Berry, *J. Hered.*, **40**, 297 (1949).
[4] Kirby, D. R. S., *Nature*, **194**, 785 (1962).
[5] Simmons, R. L., and P. S. Russell, *Nature*, **208**, 698 (1965).
[6] Kirby, D. R. S., W. D. Billingham, and D. A. James, *Transplantation*, **4**, 713 (1966).
[7] James, D. A. *Transplantation*, **8**, 846 (1969).
[8] Heyner, S., R. L. Brinster, and J. Palm, *Nature*, **222**, 783 (1969).
[9] Kirby, D. R. S., *Transplantation*, **6**, 1005 (1968).
[10] Baranska, W., and H. Koprowski, *J. Exp. Zool.*, **174**, 1 (1970).
[11] Graham, C. F., in "Heterospecific Genome Interaction," *The Wistar Institute Symposium Monograph No. 9*, ed. V. Defendi (1969), p. 19.
[12] Brinster, R. L., *J. Exp. Zool.*, **158**, 49 (1965).
[13] Wu, J. T., and R. K. Meyer, *Proc. Soc. Exp. Biol. Med.*, **123**, 88 (1966).
[14] Mintz, B., *Science*, **138**, 594 (1962).
[15] Häyry, P., and V. Defendi, *Virology*, **41**, 22 (1970).
[16] Todaro, G. J., H. Green, and B. D. Goldberg, *Proc. Nat. Acad. Sci. USA*, **51**, 66 (1964).
[17] Bodmer, W. F., M. B. Tripp, and J. A. Bodmer, in *Histocompatibility Testing*, eds. E. S. Curtoni, P. L. Mattiuz, and R. M. Tisi (1967), p. 341.
[18] Hellström, I., and H. O. Sjögren, *Exp. Cell Res.*, **40**, 212 (1965).
[19] Möller, G., *J. Exp. Med.*, **114**, 415 (1961).
[20] Pearson, G., and G. Freeman, *Cancer Res.*, **28**, 1665 (1968).
[21] Burger, M. M., *Proc. Nat. Acad. Sci. USA*, **62**, 994 (1969).
[22] Abelev, G. I., *Acta Unio Internationalis Contra Cancrum*, **19**, 80 (1963).
[23] Gold, P., and S. O. Freedman, *J. Exp. Med.*, **122**, 467 (1965).
[24] Prehn, R. T., in *Cross-reacting Antigens and Neoantigens*, ed. J. Trentin (Baltimore: Williams and Wilkins Co., 1967), p. 105.
[25] Tatarinov, Y. S., *Fed. Proc.*, **25**, T344 (1966), (translation supplement).

Cutaneous skin test for delayed hypersensitivity in hamsters to viral induced tumor antigens[1]

Richard G. Olsen, James R. McCammon, Joseph Weber, and David S. Yohn

The cell-mediated immune response is now recognized by many investigators (1) as playing a determining role in the hosts immunologic defense against oncogenesis. In vitro means to monitor cell-mediated immunity have included macrophage inhibition (3), cytotoxicity (7), and colony inhibition (4). These procedures have not always correlated with in vivo observations. Consequently many studies continue to rely on specific delayed-type hypersensitivity reactions in vivo (2, 5).

Since the hamster is commonly used as a model system in experimental viral oncology it was of interest to determine whether a similar specific skin test response could be monitored in this laboratory animal to DNA and RNA virus induced tumor antigens.

The hamster tumors used in this study were induced with adenovirus type-12 (Ad-12), Rous Sarcoma Virus, Schmidt-Rupin strain (RSV-SR), and SV40 virus or SV40 DNA. The Ad-12 tumors were from a transplantable line described previously (9). The RSV-SR tumors were transplanted at 3- to 4-week intervals in weanling PD-4 inbred hamsters, while primary SV40 tumors were induced in random bred hamsters. For preparation of skin test antigens, RSV-SR tumors were homogenized in an equal volume of Hanks' balanced salt solution (H-BSS), clarified by centrifugation, and subsequently precipitated with 2 M neutral ammonium sulphate. The precipitate was dissolved in distilled water and dialyzed against distilled water. The final preparation contained about 16 units of COFAL antigen per milliliter and about 4.6 mg protein/ml.

Ad-12 transplantable tumors and SV-40 primary tumors were freed of necrotic material, washed, minced finely, and placed in equal volume of H-BSS. This material was subsequently sonicated in an ice bath at 20 kc/s for 4 min. The Ad-12 preparation contained about 64 units of complement-fixing T-antigen per milliliter and about 42 mg protein/ml.

Skin test procedure consisted of removing the hair by shaving followed by skin testing intradermally with 0.05 ml of appropriate antigens. Skin tests were considered positive if they developed 16–48 h postinoculation and if the erythema and induration were larger than 4.0 mm. The gross appearance and histopathology of the positive skin tests in hamsters were similar to that described by Ramseier and Billingham (6).

In the RSV-SR, Ad-12, and SV-40 tumor systems the immunologic specificity of the skin test was determined by testing tumor-bearing hamsters with homologous and heterologous tumor antigens simultaneously.

[1]This study was supported in part by National Institutes of Health Contract No. 69-2233 from the Special Virus Cancer Program of the National Cancer Institute.

Of 39 Ad-12 tumor bearing inbred hamsters, 36 reacted to Ad-12 tumor antigen and none to SV-40 tumor antigens (Table 1). One of 16 Ad-12 tumor bearing hamsters tested reacted with RSV-SR tumor antigen whereas balanced salt solution failed to elicit a positive skin test in these animals.

Of 77 inbred hamsters bearing RSV-SR tumors 60 gave a positive delayed-type skin test to RSV-SR tumor antigens. In this group only 1 out of 77 cross-reacted with Ad-12 antigen and none reacted with balanced salt solution control antigen.

Skin tests on non-tumor bearing hamsters revealed no reaction with Ad-12 tumor antigens in 25 animals tested; no reaction in 10 animals tested with SV-40 antigens and no reaction in 17 animals tested with balanced salt solution. RSV-SR antigens gave a false positive response in one of the seven non-tumor bearing animals.

The skin test was used to determine the onset of delayed-type immune response following tumor challenge. Ad-12 and RSV-SR tumor bearing hamsters developed positive delayed-type skin test to homologous antigen at the time tumors became palpable (Table 2). The earliest positive skin test appeared two weeks after inoculation with tumor. All but one positive animal converted by the fifth or sixth week. With one exception the non-tumor-bearing control hamsters that were skin-tested each week remained negative during the 6-week experimental period, demonstrating that the skin test antigen did not readily sensitize the animals.

No generalization can be made about the extent of the skin test response and the size of tumor in either the RSV or Ad-12 experiments. It should be emphasized, however, that the skin test response did not diminish as the tumor increased in mass. Rats with tumors, induced by benzypyrene (8), developed a positive skin test only if macroscopic amounts of tumor were removed; thus it was proposed that the immune response was exhausted by large tumor masses.

The use of inbred hamsters in our experiments precluded the possibility of histocompatibility reactions. The absence of a positive skin test by Ad-12 and RSV-SR tumor bearing hamsters to SV40 tumor antigen, which was prepared from tumors induced in random bred hamsters,

TABLE 1

Delayed-type hypersensitivity reactions induced in the skin of hamsters bearing virus-induced transplanted tumors

Source of skin test antigen	Delayed-type hypersensitivity skin reactions in hamsters with:			
	Ad-12 tumor	RSV-SR tumor	SV-40 tumor	No tumor
Ad-12 hamster tumor (PD-4)	36/39[a]	1/77	0/8	0/25
RSV-SR hamster tumor (PD-4)	1/16	60/77	n.t.	1/7
SV-40 hamster tumor (random-bred)	0/39	n.t.	4/8	0/10
Control-balanced salt solution	0/16	0/77	0/8	0/17

[a] Number positive over number tested.
NOTE: n.t. = not tested.

TABLE 2

Time course of development of delayed-type hypersensitivity in hamsters to tumor antigens found in Ad-12 and Rous virus induced transplantable tumors

Weeks after tumor transplantation	Positive delayed-type skin reactions/number of hamsters with tumors/ number of hamsters transplanted with		No tumor (controls) but skin tested with:	
	Ad-12 tumor	RSV-SR tumor	Ad-12 Ag	RSV-SR Ag
0	0/0/5	0/0/9	0/0/5	0/0/4
1	0/0/5	0/0/9	0/0/5	0/0/4
2	2/1/5	n.t.	0/0/5	n.t.
3	3/3/5	4/5/9	0/0/5	0/0/4
4	4/4/5	n.t.	0/0/5	n.t.
5	5/5/5	n.t.	0/0/5	n.t.
6	5/5/5	6/7/7	1/0/5	0/0/4

further indicates that histocompatibility antigens were not responsible for these reactions.

The nature of the antigens in the RSV and Ad-12 systems which elicited the positive skin test response is uncertain. The Ad-12 tumor contained T-antigen and tumor specific transplantation antigen (TSTA). The RSV tumor contained avian leukosis group specific antigens; TSTA antigens were probably present. Experiments are being conducted to ascertain whether the skin test can be used to detect a response to Ad-12 TSTA antigens.

1. ALLISON, H. D. 1967. Cell mediated immune responses to virus infections and virus induced tumors. Brit. Med. Bull. 23: 60–65.
2. CHURCHILL, W. H., JR., H. U. RAPP, B. S. KRONMAN, and T. BORSOS. 1968. Detection of antigens of a new diethylnitrosomine-induced transplantable hepatoma by delayed hypersensitivity. J. Nat. Cancer Inst. 41: 13–29.
3. GEORGE, M., and J. H. VAUGHN. 1962. In vitro cell migration as a model for delayed hypersensitivity. Proc. Soc. Exp. Biol. Med. 11: 514.
4. HELLSTRÖM, I. 1967. A colony inhibition (CT) technique for demonstration of tumor cell destruction by lymphoid cells in vitro. Int. J. Cancer, 2: 65–68.
5. HOLLINSHEAD, A., D. GLEN, B. BUNNAG, P. GOLD, and R. HERBERMAN. 1970. Skin-reactive soluble antigen from intestinal cancer-cell membranes and relationship to carcinoembryonic antigens. Lancet, 6: 1191–1195.
6. RAMSEIER, J., and R. E. BILLINGHAM. 1964. Delayed cutaneous hypersensitivity reactions and transplantation immunity in syrian hamster. Ann. N.Y. Acad. Sci. 120: 379–392.
7. RUDDLE, N. H., and B. H. WAKSMAN. 1967. Cytotoxic effect of lymphocyte-antigen interaction in delayed hypersensitivity. Science (Washington), 157: 1060.
8. WANG, M. 1968. Delayed hypersensitivity to extracts from primary sarcomata in the autochthonous host. Int. J. Cancer, 3: 483–490.
9. YOHN, D. S., L. WEISS, and M. E. NEIDERS. 1968. A comparison of the distribution of tumors produced by intravenous injection of type 12 Adenovirus and Adeno-12 tumor cells. Cancer Res. 28: 571–576.

Further Studies on Loss of T-Antigen from Somatic Hybrids between Mouse Cells and SV40-Transformed Human Cells*

Mary C. Weiss

Introduction. Mammalian cells transformed by the small DNA-containing papovavirus SV40 usually do not produce infectious virus, but they do contain the complete virus genome. This can be demonstrated by fusing transformed cells with susceptible indicator (green monkey kidney) cells; the fusion products often release infectious virus.[1] SV40-transformed cells also contain a new antigen, the nuclear T-antigen,[2] which is thought to be the product of a viral gene.

We have used somatic hybrids between human and mouse cells to investigate the relationship between the viral genome and the cell it has transformed. These hybrids represent favorable material for such a study because they undergo extensive and rapid loss of human chromosomes.[3] Hybrids made between mouse cells and SV40-transformed human cells rapidly lose the chromosomes of the transformed (human) parent, and thus permit one to establish whether there is a correlation between the loss of human chromosomes and the loss of the SV40-induced T-antigen. A positive correlation between these two events would suggest that the virus genome is present in association with the chromosomes of the transformed cell rather than as a free (either nuclear or cytoplasmic) particle.

A previous publication[4] gave the first results of this study. It will be recalled that two crosses were made between mouse cells and SV40-transformed human cells; the hybrids (designated HM-SV and VT) were studied over a period of more than 100 cell generations to determine the number of human chromosomes

69

present and the presence or absence of T-antigen. It was found that the young HM-SV hybrids (about 20 generations old) contained T-antigen and 5–10 human chromosomes; similarly, the young VT hybrids contained T-antigen, but nearly 20 human chromosomes. After further growth, many cells of the former hybrids lost T-antigen, and clonal analysis showed that the T-antigen negative cells contained only 0–3 human chromosomes. However, although the VT hybrids also gave rise to a few T-antigen negative cells, it proved impracticable to isolate clones of such cells; moreover, none of the clones examined contained fewer than 8 human chromosomes.

These results are consistent with the hypothesis of chromosomal integration of the SV40 genome.[4] However, an alternative interpretation is that the hybrid cells lost some cellular gene required for expression of the viral genome. A further test of the chromosomal integration hypothesis therefore requires that the T-antigen negative hybrids be made to produce T-antigen upon reinfection with SV40, and this could not be clearly demonstrated owing to the high degree of resistance of the particular mouse parental cell used in the first cross to SV40 infection. Therefore new hybrids have been made using as the mouse parental cell the contact-inhibited line 3T3,[5] which is highly susceptible to SV40 infection and transformation.[6] Moreover, more detailed karyological studies have been made of the previously described hybrids, as well as of the new ones, to determine whether there is a single human chromosome, the loss of which is invariably correlated with the conversion of hybrid cells from T-antigen positive (T$^+$) to T-antigen negative (T$^-$).[7]

Methods and Results. Table 1 shows all of the crosses which have been used in this study. The isolation of hybrids HM-SV and VT has been described previously.[4] The third cross was between VA-2, a human cell line transformed by SV40, and the mouse line 3T3. Hybrids were obtained from ultraviolet-inactivated Sendai virus-treated[8, 9] suspensions of mixtures of these two cell lines. VA-2 is resistant to 8-azaguanine[4] and 3T3 to 5-bromodeoxyuridine;[10] neither cell type can grow in medium containing hypoxanthine, aminopterin, and thymidine.[11] The hybrids, however, proliferate in this medium owing to complementation for the enzyme deficiencies of the parental cells. Hybrid colonies were observed at a frequency of one per 5×10^2 to 1×10^3 parental cells. Eighteen hybrid colonies were isolated and examined karyologically; two were selected for further study (3V-3 and 3V-15).

TABLE 1. *Mean chromosome numbers of parental and hybrid cells.**

Parental Lines†		Hybrid Lines†		
SV40-Transformed human	Mouse		No. of human	No. of mouse
		Total no.		
SV-SD-C‡:80	C1 1D‡:52	HM-SV-1‡: 58.7	5.2	53.5
VA-2‡ :71	T6‡ :40	VT-2‡ : 96.0	18.0	78.0
		VT-7‡ : 97.5	19.2	78.3
VA-2‡ :71	3T3-4E:70	3V-3 :151.5	15.8	135.7
		3V-15 :144.2	14.2	130.0

* The karyotypes of the parental and hybrid cells are described in more detail in ref. 7.
† All cell lines shown, with the exception of T6, are clones.
‡ Origin of line described in ref. 4.

The hybrid clones, when first examined at *ca.* 20 generations, contained only 15–20 human chromosomes, instead of the expected 71. With continued growth, further loss of human chromosomes was observed; this occurred most rapidly before 50 generations, and more slowly thereafter.[12] The loss of human chromosomes from one hybrid clone is shown in Figure 1.

When first examined, both 3V hybrid clones contained only T$^+$ cells, as determined by the immunofluorescent method[13] used in the first experiments.[4] However after continued propagation, T$^-$ cells appeared in the populations at 75 and 102 generations in the cases of 3V15 and 3V3, respectively. After 135 generations of growth of the 3V15 hybrids, when about half of the cells were T$^-$, 15 subclones were isolated and characterized as to karyotype and T-antigen. More than half of these subclones were found to be pure populations of T$^-$ cells, and the remainder were found to be composed of T$^+$ cells. Analysis of the karyotypes of the T$^+$ and the T$^-$ subclones, all isolated at the same time, showed that the former contained more human chromosomes than the latter (see Fig. 1).

These results confirm those previously reported for a different cross (see Table 1, IIM-SV hybrids), namely, that hybrids of mouse cells and SV40-transformed human cells are T$^+$, and that loss of this virus-induced antigen is observed only when most of the human chromosomes are lost.[4]

One of the T$^-$ subclones shown on Figure 1, 3V-15-1, which is characterized by the presence of 5 to 7 human chromosomes, was reinfected with SV40 to determine whether such hybrids, which have lost the SV40-induced T-antigen and presumably the complete virus genome, remain capable of the synthesis of T-antigen.

Confluent cultures of 3V-15-1, and of the parental 3T3 cells, were infected with SV40 as described by Todaro and Green;[14] after infection, the cells were

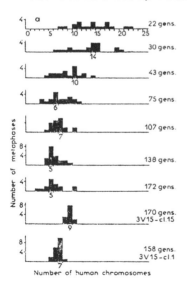

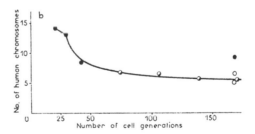

F$_{IG}$. 1.—Loss of human chromosomes from hybrid clone 3V-15. (*a*) Histogram showing the mode and the range of the numbers of human chromosomes present after different numbers of cell generations. (*b*) Curve showing the mean numbers of human chromosomes of the same hybrid clone (3V15), plotted against the number of cell generations through which the hybrid cells have grown. The presence or absence of T-antigen is indicated by the points: (●) all cells positive; (◑) mixed population; (○) all cells negative. The points which do not fall on the curve represent subclones of 3V15.

transferred to cover slips for T-antigen assay after 48 and 72 hours. T+ cells were found in the 3V-15-1 cultures at both times examined, and their frequency was 5–15%, the same as that observed for the 3T3 cells. In neither case was there a detectable cytopathic effect.

Since it appears that loss of the T-antigen occurs in conjunction with that of human chromosomes, an attempt was made to determine whether disappearance of this antigen can be linked with that of the human chromosome which specifies thymidine kinase. This human marker was selected because two of the mouse parental lines lack this enzyme, and the human enzyme activity is selected *for* in medium containing hypoxanthine, aminopterin, and thymidine (HAT) but can be selected *against* by growing hybrid cells in medium containing 5-bromo-deoxyuridine (BUdR).[3]

The HM-SV and 3V hybrids (see Table 1) were tested for T-antigen while continuously maintained in HAT, as well as after growth in BUdR. T⁻ cells appeared in all of the populations maintained in HAT medium. From this observation it can be concluded that the two independently transformed human parental lines, SV-SD-C and VA-2, contained at least one homolog of the thymidine kinase chromosome which was not associated with the SV40 genome. Moreover, populations which were T+ or mixed were not composed of T⁻ survivors after treatment with BUdR. Thus, it is clear that the human chromosome which specifies thymidine kinase[15, 16] does not contain a unique integration site for SV40.

Comparisons have been made of the karyotypes of T+ and T⁻ clones of HM-SV and 3V hybrids. The HM-SV hybrids were particularly favorable for this study since three T+ subclones were obtained which contained only 2–4 human chromosomes. All three subclones, which had been continuously maintained in

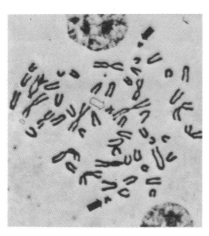

FIG. 2.—Metaphase figure of a T⁻ subclone (clone 3) of HM-SV. In metaphases of this subclone, three human chromosomes can be identified: one of Group E (*white arrow*) and two of Group G (*black arrows*).

HAT, retained the Group E chromosome which specifies thymidine kinase, and from all of them, T⁻ subclones were isolated in HAT medium, thereby showing that the thymidine kinase chromosome did not carry the SV40 genome(s). In addition, all three T+ subclones contained one or more small acrocentric Group G chromosomes (Fig. 2). Since these Group G chromosomes were the only human chromosomes retained by all of them, it seemed likely that one or more chromosomes of this group carry the SV40 genome(s). In order to confirm these observations, the T+ and T⁻ 3V15 clones and subclones were examined to determine whether Group G chromosomes would be found only in the positive ones. However, it was found that chromosomes of this group were rare in the T$^+$ clones. Moreover, T$^+$ and T$^-$ subclones of the 3V15 hybrids were found to retain human chromosomes of the same groups (A, C, E, and F), and these chromosomes were simply more numerous in the positive subclones. It seems unlikely, therefore, that there is only one human chromosome containing a specific integration site for SV40. These results are consistent with the hypothesis that different chromosomes may carry SV40 genomes in the independently transformed human parental cells, SV-SD-C and VA-2.

In addition to the detailed karyotypic analysis performed on the HM-SV and 3V15 hybrids, determinations have been made of the numbers of human chromosomes in T$^+$ and mixed hybrid clones (3V3, VT-2, and VT-7). Table 2 shows that four out of five hybrid clones gave rise to T$^-$ cells and that it was possible to isolate T$^-$ subclones from only two of these four. (Since there was no method of selecting for T$^-$ cells, isolation of T$^-$ subclones required that these cells constitute a sizable fraction of the total population.) The minimum mean number of human chromosomes observed in the hybrid clone VT-2 was 11.1, and in this population no T$^-$ cells were observed. In two others, VT-7 and 3V3, minimum mean numbers of human chromosomes of 8.4 and 8.8 were observed; in these populations, T$^-$ cells were detected, but among 15 subclones isolated from each, none were T-antigen negative. And, finally, the two hybrid populations from which T$^-$ clones were isolated contained only 1.9 and 5.6 human chromosomes after more than 150 generations (Table 2), and at this time were composed predominantly of T$^-$ cells. Table 3 shows the numbers of human

TABLE 2. *Detection and isolation of T-antigen negative cells from the different hybrid clones.*

Hybrid clone	T$^-$ cells detected	T$^-$ clones isolated	Minimum mean no.* of human chromosomes
HM-SV	Yes	Yes	1.9
VT-2	No	No	11.1
VT-7	Yes	No	8.4
3V3	Yes	No	8.8
3V15	Yes	Yes	5.6

* Minimum mean number of human chromosomes observed in hybrid clones continuously maintained in selective medium.

TABLE 3. *Number of human chromosomes of T$^+$ and T$^-$ hybrid cells.*

Hybrid	When T$^-$ First Observed No. of generations	When T$^-$ First Observed No. of human chromosomes	Characteristics of Clones No. of generations	No. of Human Chromosomes T$^+$	No. of Human Chromosomes T$^-$
HM-SV	30	5.2 (2–10)			
Clone 3			60	2.9 (2–4)	
Clone 3–8			120		1.0 (1)
Clone 6			60	2.1 (1–3)	
Clone 6–1			120	2.0 (2)	
Clone 6–3			120		1.0 (1)
VT 7	100	10.1 (2–17)			
3V3	102	8.6 (5–11)			
3V15	75	6.9 (3–11)			
3V15–1			158		6.5 (5–7)
3V15–9			158		5 (5)
3V15–15			170	9.0 (8–10)	

chromosomes present in these various populations when T$^-$ cells were first detected, as well as those of the T$^+$ and T$^-$ subclones isolated from them.

In all of these hybrids, there is a clear negative correlation between the numbers of human chromosomes and the presence, as well as the frequency, of T$^-$ cells. These results give strong support to the hypothesis of association between the chromosomes of the transformed cell and the SV40 genome.

Discussion. A different kind of experimental evidence has suggested that the SV40 genome is integrated into the chromosomes of the transformed cell. Westphal and Dulbecco[17] have hybridized labeled complementary RNA (synthesized *in vitro* from purified SV40 DNA) with DNA from SV40-transformed cells. The amount of hybridization obtained indicated the presence of multiple virus genomes in transformed cells. Moreover, Sambrook *et al.*[18] found that the hybridizable DNA from SV40-transformed mouse cells is of high molecular weight and is found only in the nucleus. They further showed that the SV40 DNA in transformed cells is covalently linked to the large molecules of cellular DNA.

The observation that there are multiple SV40 genomes in transformed cells integrated into chromosomal DNA clearly poses the question of the number of sites of integration. All genomes could be integrated in tandem into one chromosome, or they could be scattered among the chromosomes.[18] Our results are more consistent with the latter hypothesis. The T$^-$ subclones of HM-SV hybrids retained at most only one or two human chromosomes. Thus in this case, nearly every human chromosome was lost from the hybrid cells before loss of T-antigen was observed. This could mean that many of the chromosomes of the parental human cells contained SV40 genomes, or that a single human chromosome carried all of the genomes, and that its presence conferred a selective advantage upon the hybrid cells and therefore was lost nonrandomly and rather infrequently. However in mixed populations of T$^+$ and T$^-$ cells the former did not have a selective advantage; rather, the mixed populations evolved rapidly in the other direction.

The results observed with the 3V hybrids are less clear; T$^-$ subclones have been obtained which contain as many as seven human chromosomes. The human parent of this hybrid may contain fewer SV40 genomes than that of the HM-SV hybrids; this would not be unexpected since Westphal and Dulbecco[17] have observed between 5 and 60 SV40 genomes per cell in independently transformed lines. On the other hand, the VA-2 parent may contain SV40 genomes on fewer chromosomes.

The studies with hybrid cells indicate a remarkable degree of stability of the integrated virus genomes. All hybrids which have lost most or all of the human chromosomes have lost T-antigen. If the viral genomes were periodically dissociated from one chromosome and reintegrated into another, one might expect to observe hybrid cells which have lost most or all human chromosomes and still retain T-antigen, because of integration of SV40 genomes into (the much more numerous) mouse chromosomes of the hybrid cells; this has not been observed in these hybrid populations studied for more than 150 cell generations.

Marin and Littlefield[19] have studied hamster-hamster hybrid cells transformed by polyoma virus; in this case also a positive correlation was found between loss of chromosomes and loss of the polyoma genomes.

Thus the genomes of two of the small DNA-containing viruses, SV40 and polyoma, appear to be stably integrated into the chromosomes of transformed cells. Each of these viruses produces, upon transformation, a characteristic alteration of cell morphology, and the change is a permanent one, although rare revertants do appear (cf. ref. 20). It has been postulated that there is a specific viral gene which produces the alteration of cell morphology known as the "transformed phenotype." Moreover, in view of the persistence of the viral genome, it is tempting to postulate that the continuous expression of such a gene is required to maintain the transformed phenotype.

If this hypothesis were correct, one would expect the 3V (3T3 × VA-2) hybrids to express the transformed phenotype, since (1) the SV40-transformed parent contributed SV40 genomes, and (2) SV40 transformation of 3T3 causes a dramatic change in the morphology and growth characteristics of 3T3. Contrary to expectation, all 18 (3V) hybrid clones showed morphology and growth characteristics very similar to those of the 3T3 parental cells.

3T3 cells are contact inhibited; when a confluent monolayer is formed, they cease dividing. At this saturation density, the number of cells present in the monolayer remains constant over several weeks, in spite of renewals of medium. By contrast, SV40-transformed 3T3 reaches a density 10 times higher than normal 3T3 and the cells form multiple layers on the plate. The saturation density is not constant since the cells continue to grow when nutrients are provided. The saturation densities of 3T3, SV40-transformed 3T3, VA-2, and several 3V hybrid clones are shown in Table 4.

The 3T3-like growth properties of the hybrid cells were stable, and the two clones studied in detail showed little change over more than 100 generations of growth. However, from these two hybrid populations, rare variant subclones have been isolated which reach much higher saturation densities.[21] T-antigen analyses of some of these subclones have shown that there is no predictable relationship between growth properties of the cells and presence of the virus genome; some clones of this type are T+ and others are T−. The same is true of low saturation-density clones.

These observations show that the mere presence of SV40 genomes, integrated into human chromosomes and introduced into 3T3 by hybridization, does not cause the same modification in growth properties of 3T3 cells as is produced when 3T3 cells are infected, and subsequently transformed, by SV40 virus.

It is possible that these hybrid cells contain too few virus genomes to effect the transformed phenotype: even the young hybrid cells contained only 15–20

TABLE 4. Saturation densities of parental and hybrid cells.

Cell line	T-antigen	Saturation density (cells/cm²)
3T3	−	4×10^4
SV40-transformed 3T3	+	46×10^4*
VA-2	+	30×10^4
Hybrid clones (3T3 × VA-2)		
3V3	+	3×10^4
3V5	+	4.5×10^4
3V15	+	3.9×10^4
3V15-1	−	4×10^4

* Value quoted from ref. 20.

75

VA-2 chromosomes, and possibly only few SV40 genomes. On the other hand, it may be that the transformed phenotype is the consequence of some event which occurs *at the time* of transformation, and cannot be effected by virus genomes once they have become integrated into the chromosomes of the transformed cell.

The question whether there is a viral gene, the continuous activity of which is required to maintain the transformed phenotype, is at present being investigated by the study of temperature-sensitive mutants of polyoma virus.[22] If there is such a viral gene, it should be possible to find mutants and obtain cell transformants which express the transformed phenotype only at a permissive temperature, and a normal phenotype at a nonpermissive temperature which does not allow expression of the "transforming" gene.

I thank Dr. Boris Ephrussi for his continued interest in this work, for many stimulating discussions, and for his critical reading of the manuscript. I am indebted to Melle Anne Debon for her excellent technical assistance.

Abbreviations used: T^+ (T-antigen positive); T^- (T-antigen negative); HAT (selective medium containing hypoxanthine, aminopterin, and thymidine); BUdR (5-bromodeoxyuridine).

* This work was conducted with the aid of USPHS postdoctoral fellowship F2-GM-34,679 at the Carnegie Institution of Washington, Department of Embryology, and at the Centre de Génétique Moléculaire du Centre National de la Recherche Scientifique with the help of the Délégation Générale à la Recherche Scientifique et Technique.

[1] Koprowski, H., F. C. Jensen, and Z. Steplewski, these PROCEEDINGS, 58, 127 (1967); Watkins, J. F., and R. Dulbecco, these PROCEEDINGS, 58, 1396 (1967).

[2] Black, P. H., W. P. Rowe, H. C. Turner, and R. J. Huebner, these PROCEEDINGS, 50, 1148 (1963).

[3] Weiss, M. C., and H. Green, these PROCEEDINGS, 58, 1104 (1967).

[4] Weiss, M. C., B. Ephrussi, and L. J. Scaletta, these PROCEEDINGS, 59, 1132 (1968).

[5] Todaro, G. J., and H. Green, J. Cell Biol., 17, 299 (1963).

[6] Todaro, G. J., and H. Green, Virology, 23, 117 (1964).

[7] A more complete report of these experiments will appear in: Weiss, M. C., "Genetic Concepts and Neoplasia," in 23rd Annual Symposium on Fundamental Cancer Research, 1969 (Baltimore: Williams and Wilkins, in press).

[8] Harris, H., and J. F. Watkins, Nature, 205, 640 (1965).

[9] Coon, H. G., and M. C. Weiss, these PROCEEDINGS, 62, 852 (1969).

[10] Matsuya, Y., and H. Green, Science, 163, 697 (1969).

[11] Littlefield, J. W., Science, 145, 709 (1964).

[12] All estimates of numbers of parental chromosomes in somatic hybrids must be made with the reservation that translocations and other chromosomal rearrangements can and almost certainly do occur.

[13] Pope, J. H., and W. P. Rowe, J. Exptl. Med., 120, 121 (1964); Rapp, F., J. S. Butel, and J. L. Melnick, Proceedings of the Society for Experimental Biology, 116, 1131 (1964).

[14] Todaro, G. J., and H. Green, Virology, 28, 756 (1966).

[15] Migeon, B., and C. Miller, Science, 162, 1005 (1968).

[16] Matsuya, H., H. Green, and C. Basilico, Nature, 220, 1199 (1968).

[17] Westphal, H., and R. Dulbecco, these PROCEEDINGS, 59, 1158 (1968).

[18] Sambrook, J., H. Westphal, P. R. Srinivasan, and R. Dulbecco, these PROCEEDINGS, 60, 1288 (1968).

[19] Marin, G., and J. W. Littlefield, J. Virology, 2, 69 (1968).

[20] Pollack, R. E., H. Green, and G. J. Todaro, these PROCEEDINGS, 60, 126 (1968).

[21] Similar results have been obtained from crosses of 3T3 with mouse L cells; Weiss, M. C., G. J. Todaro, and H. Green, J. Cell. Physiol., 71, 105 (1968).

[22] Eckhart, W., Virology, 38, 120 (1969); Di Mayorca, G., J. Callender, G. Marin, and R. Giordano, Virology, 38, 126 (1969).

Comparison of Transformation and T Antigen Induction in Human Cell Lines

C. W. POTTER, A. M. POTTER, AND J. S. OXFORD

Simian virus 40 (SV40) has been shown to transform hamster, mouse, rabbit, monkey, and rat cells in tissue culture [reviewed by Black (2)]. In addition, in vitro transformation of human cells has been reported by several workers (6, 16) and the frequency of transformation was quantitatively measured (17). Studies of cell cultures from patients with Down's syndrome (18) and Franconi's anaemia (17) have shown these cells to be more susceptible to transformation by SV40 virus than cells from normal individuals: both these diseases are known to be associated with a high incidence of natural malignancies (3). An extension of these studies might be of value in the identification of persons with relatively high susceptibility to certain malignant diseases (7).

The incidence of SV40 virus-induced T antigen (4) in dividing cell cultures of human cells has been reported to relate directly to their susceptibility to transformation by SV40 virus (1). In the present study, both dividing and nondividing cell cultures, showing different transformation frequencies, were examined for the presence of SV40 virus-induced T antigen. In addition, the incidence of T antigen induced by chick embryo lethal orphan (CELO) virus, a second virus tumorigenic for hamsters (15), was calculated for a number of cell lines. The susceptibility of the cell lines to infection by two additional viruses, vaccinia virus and influenza virus A2/Scotland/49/57, which have not been shown to produce tumors in laboratory animals, is also reported.

MATERIALS AND METHODS

Cell cultures. Human fibroblast cultures were derived from skin specimens, cut into several small fragments, and anchored in glass vessels with human plasma clots (5). The cultures were grown in Eagle's basal medium (EBM) containing 10% fetal bovine serum (Flow Laboratories Inc., Irvine, Scotland), 10% tryptose phosphate broth, and antibiotics (100 units/ml of penicillin and 100 μg/ml of streptomycin). The growth medium was changed at intervals of 3 to 4 days, and confluent monolayers were obtained after 14 to 28 days of incubation at 37 C. Fully grown cultures of cells were passaged at 1:2 dilution at intervals of 4 to 6 days. All tests were carried out at the 5th to 10th in vitro passage. Human fibroblast cells (W1-38) were obtained at the 25th passage level and were subcultured at intervals of 4 to 6 days by using the same methods as described for other human cell lines. W1-38 cells were tested for transformation frequency and susceptibility to T antigen induction at the 26th to 30th passage.

African green monkey kidney cells (Flow Laboratories Inc.) were grown in medium 199 containing 5% calf serum, 0.44 g per liter of sodium bicarbonate and antibiotics. The cells were maintained in medium 199 containing 2% calf serum and 0.88 g per liter of sodium bicarbonate. BHK21 cells were grown in EBM containing 10% inactivated calf serum, 10% tryptose phosphate broth, and antibiotics, and maintained in the same medium modified to contain 2% calf serum.

Chromosome analysis. Human fibroblast cells were subcultured, at a concentration to give 50% confluent cell sheets after 36 hr of incubation, in medium 199 containing 20% fetal bovine serum and 20% tryptose phosphate broth. After 36 hr of incubation, colcemid (CIBA Laboratories Ltd., Horsham, Sussex) was added to a final concentration of 0.02 μg/ml, and the cultures were further incubated for 4 to 6 hr. After incubation, the cells were washed with phosphate-buffered saline (PBS), detached from the culture vessels by using 0.25% trypsin, and swollen by the addition of an equal volume of distilled water. The cells were fixed in acetic acid-ethyl alcohol (1:3), spread on grease-free, wet, ice-cold slides, air-dried, and stained with 2% aceto-orcein.

Chromosome counts were performed on 30 well-spread metaphase figures, and a further four cells were analyzed to establish the cell karyotype. In one specimen (M16), which proved to be a mosaic of two cell types, chromosome counts were performed on 80 cells, and the karyotype was established from an analysis of a further 20 cells.

Viruses. Primary monolayer cultures of AGMK cells were infected with SV40 virus, obtained from A. J. Girardi, Wistar Institute of Anatomy and Biology, Philadelphia, Pa., at a concentration of 0.1 TCD_{50}/cell. When cytopathic effect was complete, cultures were frozen and thawed twice (−80 C/22 C), and centrifuged at 2,000 × g for 20 min, and the supernatant fluids were stored in 5- to 10-ml volumes at −80 C. The titer of this virus preparation after 21 days of incubation in AGMK cells was $10^{8.3} TCD_{50}$/ml (14).

The Phelps strain of CELO virus (11) was used to inoculate the allantoic cavity of 7-day chick embryos. After 3 days of incubation at 36 C, the allantoic fluids were harvested, pooled, and stored at −20 C. This virus pool had a titer of $10^{9.2}$ TCD_{50}/ml in cultures of chick kidney cells (8).

Influenza virus A2/Scotland/49/57 was obtained from the allantoic fluids of 10-day embryonated eggs inoculated with 10^{-3} dilution of stock virus and incubated at 35 C for 48 hr. A pool of vaccinia virus was obtained from virus-infected BHK21 cells. Cultures showing complete cytopathic effect were frozen and thawed once (−80 C/22 C) and centrifuged at 2,000 × g for 20 min, and the supernatant fluids were stored at −80 C.

Transformation studies. The transformation frequency of human cells was measured by the technique of Todaro et al. (17). Eight to 12 cultures were used for each cell line tested, and the transformation frequency was expressed as the percentage of SV40 virus-infected cells forming transformed foci.

Induction of T antigen. Human fibroblast cells were inoculated into 50-mm petri dishes containing glass cover slips at a concentration to produce confluent growth after 3 days of incubation. After this time, the nondividing cells were washed twice with Hanks' saline and inoculated with either 1.0 ml of SV40 or CELO virus. After incubation for 3 hr at 37 C, the cell sheets were washed with two changes of Hanks' saline and incubated in growth medium; for cultures infected with SV40 virus, 0.5% rabbit anti-SV40 serum

(neutralizing titer 1:512 to 1:1024) was included in the growth medium. Cover slips of infected cells were harvested after various times of incubation, washed in PBS, fixed in acetone at −20 C, air-dried, and stored at −80 C.

In further experiments, the incidence of SV40 virus-induced T antigen was estimated for dividing cells. Monolayer cultures of human fibroblasts were infected with SV40 or CELO virus and incubated for 18 hr in growth medium. The cells were then suspended with 0.25% trypsin, diluted 1:5, and inoculated into 50-mm petri dishes containing cover slips. Cover slips were harvested at various intervals, washed in acetone, air-dried, and stored at −80 C.

Cover slip preparations of infected cells were examined by the indirect immunofluorescence technique for virus-induced T antigen (12). After thawing, the cover slips were treated with a 1:4 dilution of serum from hamsters bearing large, transplanted SV40 or CELO virus-induced tumors containing complement-fixing antibody titer 1:80 and 1:40, respectively (13), washed, and stained with fluorescein-labeled goat antihamster serum (Nordic Diagnostics, Tilburg, The Netherlands). The slides were viewed with a Gillett and Sibert conference microscope illuminated with an iodine quartz light source. Percentages of cells containing T antigen were estimated from the observation of 2,000 to 4,000 cells.

Sensitivity of cell lines to infection with vaccinia virus and influenza virus A2/Scotland/49/57. Monolayer cultures of nondividing cells were washed with Hanks' saline, and infected with either vaccinia virus or influenza virus A2/Scotland/49/57. Logarithmic dilutions of a virus pool, diluted to the lowest concentration capable of infecting all cells, were used to infect cells. After 1 hr of incubation at 36 C, the cells were washed with Hanks' saline to remove unabsorbed virus and incubated for 22 hr in fresh growth medium. After incubation the cover slips were harvested, fixed in cold acetone, air dried, and stored at −80 C. The infectivity of the viruses for cells was assessed by the indirect immunofluorescence technique (9), and the results were expressed as the virus dilution which produced specific fluorescence in 50% of the cells (FD_{50}/ml).

RESULTS

Transformation frequencies. The transformation frequency was established for skin fibroblast cultures from eight individuals, and for WI-38 cells. The results are shown in Table 1. Four cell lines were grouped together as having a low susceptibility to transformation (0.017 to 0.024%). This transformation-resistant group (TR) included WI-38 cells, two cell lines from infants aged less than 1 month whose cells contained a normal chromosome complement, and cell line M29 from adult aged 26 years whose cells contained an XYY chromosome complement.

A second group of cell lines, including M21, M24, M25, and M26, were calculated to have a higher susceptibility to transformation (0.061 to

Susceptibility to transformation	Code	Age (years)	Chromosome content (sex)	Total infected cells plated	Total number of transformed foci	Transformation rate[a]
Low (TR)	WI-38		Normal (F)	5.2×10^5	88	0.017
	M 5	<1/12	Normal (M)	5.4×10^5	113	0.021
	M 20	<1/12	Normal (M)	4.4×10^5	106	0.024
	M 29	26	XYY (M)	4.7×10^5	99	0.021
Intermediate	M 16	4	95% Normal 5% Trisomy 17/18 (F)	6.1×10^5	256	0.042
High (TS)	M 21	10	Trisomy 21/22 (M)	4.3×10^5	357	0.083
	M 24	13	Trisomy 21/22 (F)	4.5×10^5	274	0.061
	M 25	12	Trisomy 21/22 (M)	6.4×10^5	441	0.069
	M 26	13	Trisomy 21/22 (M)	4.0×10^5	260	0.065

[a] Expressed as the ratio (in per cent) of total number of infected cells plated to total number of transformed foci.

0.083%). The results indicated that these cell lines (TS) were three to four times more susceptible to transformation than TR cell lines (Table 1). All the TS cell lines had been established from patients with Down's syndrome aged 10 to 13 years, and cytogenetic studies showed that the cells from all four individuals possessed trisomy for chromosomes 21/22.

A single cell line M16, established from a child aged 4 years, was found to be a mosaic, 95% of the cells contained a normal chromosome complement and 5% possessed trisomy for chromosomes 17/18. The transformation frequency for cell line M16 was established as 0.042%, and this cell line was intermediate in its susceptibility to transformation.

Although other studies have reported that cells from patients with Down's syndrome have a greater susceptibility to transformation than cells from normal persons (18), this conclusion is not allowed in the present study. The cell lines are not adequately matched (Table 1), and susceptibility to transformation may vary by age.

Induction of SV40 virus-induced T antigen. Table 2 shows the percentage of cells containing T antigen, detectable by immunofluorescence tests, in nondividing cultures of human fibroblast cells infected with SV40 virus and harvested after various times. SV40 virus-induced T antigen was detected after 24 hr of incubation of infected TR cell lines. The percentage of fluorescent-positive cells increased to a maximum of 19.7 to 30.8% after 2 to 5 days of in-

TABLE 2. *Induction of simian virus 40 T antigen in nondividing cell lines*

Susceptibility to transformation	Code	Days after virus infection					
		0	1	2	3	5	7
Low (TR)	WI-38	<0.1[a]	8.3	19.7	17.8	11.2	NT[b]
	M 5	<0.1	0.8	5.4	11.5	30.8	8.5
	M 20	<0.1	0.4	2.3	14.3	17.1	6.2
	M 29	<0.1	1.1	6.3	13.1	26.2	15.7
Intermediate	M 16	<0.1	<0.1	4.6	9.0	8.0	2.0
High (TS)	M 21	<0.1	<0.1	0.6	1.2	1.6	0.3
	M 24	<0.1	<0.1	1.3	2.0	1.8	NT
	M 25	<0.1	<0.1	1.2	1.5	0.8	0.6
	M 26	<0.1	<0.1	0.7	1.5	0.8	0.5

[a] Values expressed as percentage of cells containing T antigen.
[b] Not tested.

cubation, but later decreased. Similar studies of TS cells lines indicated that the percentage of cells with detectable SV40 virus-induced T antigen was significantly lower. Thus, SV40-induced T antigen was not observed until 48 hr after infection, and the maximum percentage of cells containing T antigen varied from 1.2 to 2.0% after 3 to 5 days of incubation.

SV40 infection of cell cultures from patient M16, a cell line containing both cells of normal chromosome content and cells with trisomy for chromosomes 17/18 and intermediate in sensitivity for transformation by SV40 virus, resulted in T antigen induction in a maximum of 9.0% of cells. This result was lower than that seen for TR cell lines and greater than found in TS cell lines.

The incidence of SV40 virus-induced T antigen in dividing cells, cells which had been plated 18 hr after virus infection, was in contrast to results obtained in nondividing cells. The findings are shown in Table 3. For TR cell lines, the maximum incidence of cells containing SV40-induced T antigen was found 3 to 4 days after virus infection, and was calculated to be 0.70 to 1.5%. A higher percentage of T antigen-containing cells was found in TS cell lines; the maximum incidence was observed 3 days after infection and was calculated to be 1.81 to 2.80%.

In further experiments, nondividing cells were plated at daily intervals for 5 days after SV40-virus infection, and the cells were fixed and stained 20 hr later. The incidence of T antigen in the plated cells was similar to that seen in unplated cells incubated for the same period of time.

Induction of CELO virus-induced T antigen. Nondividing, monolayer cultures of fibroblast cells grown on cover slips were infected with CELO virus, harvested at various intervals, and tested by the indirect immunofluorescence technique for the presence of CELO virus-induced T antigen. The results are given in Table 4. The presence of CELO virus-induced T antigen was first detected after 24 hr of incubation of infected TR cell lines, and the maximum percentage of T-antigen containing cells was found to vary from 2.26 to 4.12% after 3 days of incubation; lower percentages were observed for cultures incubated for 5 and 7 days.

TABLE 3. *Induction of simian virus 40 T antigen in dividing cell cultures*

Susceptibility to transformation	Code	Days after virus infection				
		2	3	4	6	8
Low (TR)	M 5	0.20[a]	1.04	1.50	0.62	0.44
	M 20	0.30	0.90	0.63	0.35	0.23
	W1–38	0.60	0.70	0.70	0.25	0.10
High (TS)	M 21	NT[b]	2.80	1.30	0.25	0.09
	M 25	0.30	1.81	1.22	0.62	0.31
	M 26	0.98	2.4	2.07	1.61	0.62

[a] Values are expressed as percentage cells containing T antigen.
[b] Not tested.

TABLE 4. *Induction of CELO virus T antigen in nondividing cells*

Susceptibility to transformation	Code	Days after virus infection					
		0	1	2	3	5	7
Low (TR)	W1–38	<0.01[a]	0.10	2.82	4.12	3.80	NT[b]
	M 5	<0.01	0.06	11.30	3.00	2.16	0.21
	M 20	<0.01	0.05	1.22	2.26	0.46	NT
Intermediate	M 29	<0.01	<0.01	0.45	2.31	1.82	0.51
	M 16	<0.01	<0.01	<0.01	0.20	0.30	NT
High (TS)	M 21	<0.01	<0.01	<0.01	0.01	0.12	0.02
	M 24	<0.01	<0.01	<0.01	0.08	0.05	0.08
	M 25	<0.01	<0.01	<0.01	0.11	0.08	0.05
	M 26	<0.01	<0.01	<0.01	0.10	0.05	0.01

[a] Values are expressed as percentage of cells containing T antigen.
[b] Not tested

The incidence of CELO virus induced T antigen was significantly lower in nondividing TS cells than in TR cells. TS cell lines did not show demonstrable T antigen at 48 hr after virus infection; all the cell lines contained cells with T antigen 72 hr after infection, and the maximal incidence of antigen positive cells was 0.08 to 0.12% (Table 4). The results indicated that nondividing cultures of TR cell lines were 10- to 20-fold more susceptible to induction of CELO virus T antigen than similar cultures of TS cells.

CELO virus infection of nondividing cells of cell line M16 induced virus specific T antigen in a maximum of 0.3% of cells. This result was less than found in nondividing TR cells, and greater than seen in nondividing TS cells.

The incidence of CELO virus-induced T antigen was also measured in dividing cultures of three TR and three TS cell lines. The highest incidence of fluorescent-positive cells in TR cell lines was 0.05 to 0.07%, in cells examined 3 days after plating. In only one line, M20, were T antigen-positive cells found in cultures examined 7 days after plating. The results obtained for TS cell lines were very similar; the maximum incidence of fluorescent-positive cells was 0.05 to 0.08%. Observations of TS cells 7 days after plating indicated a very low incidence ($< 0.01\%$) of fluorescent-positive cells.

Sensitivity of cell lines to infection with vaccinia virus and influenza virus A2/Scotland/49/57. Infectivity titration of vaccinia virus and influenza virus A2/Scotland/49/57 was carried out in nondividing cultures of both TR and TS cell lines. The results, expressed as FD_{50}/ml of the highest virus concentration used to infect cells, are shown in Table 5. The titer of influenza virus A/2 Scotland/49/57 for three TR cells lines was $10^{1.26}$ to $10^{1.43}$ FD_{50}/ml. These values were significantly greater than those found for the three TS

TABLE 5. *Production of influenza virus A2/Scotland/49/57 and vaccinia virus fluorescent antigens in nondividing TS and TR cell lines*

Susceptibility to transformation	Code	Percentage of fluorescing cells after infection with									
		Log_{10} dilutions of influenza virus A2/Scotland/49/57				FD_{50}/ml	Log_{10} dilutions of vaccinia virus				FD_{50}/ml
		10^0	10^{-1}	10^{-2}	10^{-3}		10^0	10^{-1}	10^{-2}	10^{-2}	
TR	M 5	100	85	7.6	1.1	$10^{1.26}$	100	35.1	3.5	0.5	$10^{0.94}$
	M 20	100	100	12.2	1.0	$10^{1.63}$	100	17.2	1.3	0.2	$10^{0.76}$
	W1-38	100	100	8.4	1.2	$10^{1.43}$	100	20.9	1.8	0.4	$10^{0.85}$
TS	M 21	100	16.3	3.4	0.3	$10^{0.78}$	100	28.2	3.6	0.6	$10^{0.86}$
	M 25	100	29.1	3.1	0.4	$10^{0.86}$	100	24.1	2.3	0.4	$10^{0.79}$
	M 26	100	23.4	2.8	0.5	$10^{0.83}$	100	15.9	1.8	0.2	$10^{0.67}$

cell lines where the titers were $10^{0.78}$ to $10^{0.85}$ FD_{50}/ml. These differences were consistently observed in multiple experiments and indicated that TR cell lines are three to five times more sensitive to infection by influenza virus A2/Scotland/49/57 than TS cells.

Titrations of vaccinia virus in nondividing cultures of TR and TS cells indicated that the cell lines were equally sensitive to vaccinia virus. Thus, the virus titer for TR cells was $10^{0.76}$ to $10^{0.94}$ FD_{50}/ml, and for TS cells was $10^{0.67}$ to $10^{0.86}$ FD_{50}/ml (Table 5).

DISCUSSION

Measurements of transformation frequency of nine human cell lines in the present study indicate considerable variation in susceptibility to virus-induced transformation. Cell lines established from four patients with Down's syndrome were found to be three to four times more susceptible to transformation than were two cell lines from infants whose cells contained a normal chromosome content, a cell line from an adult whose cells contained XYY chromosomes, and W1-38 cells. The greater susceptibility of cells from patients with Down's syndrome to transformation has been reported previously (1, 18). Of intermediate susceptibility to transformation were cells derived from a patient M16, for whom cytogenetic studies of peripheral blood cells indicated trisomy for chromosomes 17/18 in all cells. However, analysis of skin fibroblast cells showed that only 5% of cells contained trisomy 17/18 and the remainder were normal. Todaro and Martin (18) reported that cells from a single patient with trisomy 17 18 were more susceptible to transformation by SV40 virus than were cells from either normal persons or patients with Down's syndrome. The intermediate sensitivity to transformation of cells from patient M16 may be due to the low proportion of

highly susceptible, trisomy 17/18 cells in this culture.

Cell cultures exhibiting low and high susceptibility to transformation by SV40 virus were compared for T antigen induction after infection with SV40 virus. The incidence of cells containing SV40-induced T antigen depended on the technique used. When nondividing cells were infected with SV40 virus the incidence of cells containing T antigen was approximately 10-fold greater for TR cell lines than for TS cell lines. Thus, the susceptibility of nondividing cells to T antigen induction does not relate to susceptibility to SV40 virus transformation.

In contrast, for dividing cell cultures, the maximum incidence of SV40 virus-induced T antigen was 1.81 to 2.80% for three TS cell lines, derived from patients with Down's syndrome, and 0.70 to 1.5% for three TR cell lines. Repeated experiments on individual cell lines indicate that these results were reproducible to ±0.35%. Since the variation between the different TS cells was as great as the difference between TS and TR cell lines, further lines should be examined to establish clearly the significance of these findings. Aaronson and Todaro (1), who examined dividing cell cultures of SV40 virus-infected cells, showed that SV40 T antigen was detected in a greater percentage of cells from patients with Down's syndrome than in cells from normal persons.

The incidence of SV40 virus-induced T antigen in nondividing TR cell cultures was approximately 10- to 20-fold greater than observed in cultures of dividing cells. Similar results have been reported previously by Oxman and Black (10). These authors suggested that the results were due to incomplete incorporation of the virus genome into the host cell genome, and a subsequent loss of virus genome and T antigen-inducing capacity in dividing cell cultures. An alternative explana-

81

tion is that SV40 virus infection of TR cells is lethal, and many infected cells are not present in plated cultures. However, the incidence of T antigen in SV40 virus-infected cells which were plated after 1 to 5 days of incubation and examined 20 hr later indicated that cells containing demonstrable T antigen could be successfully plated.

Studies similar to those described by using SV40 virus were also carried out with CELO virus. CELO virus shares several properties with SV40 virus, including oncogenicity for newborn hamsters (15) and the induction of a specific tumour antigen (13). The results obtained for T antigen induction in the cell lines with CELO virus parallel those obtained with SV40 virus. Thus, antigen was induced in a greater proportion of nondividing TR cells than in TS cells. However, results for dividing cells indicate a very low incidence of fluorescence-positive cells for both TR and TS cells.

The relatively high susceptibility to infection of nondividing TR cell lines with SV40 and CELO virus, compared with that of TS cells, is not limited to tumorigenic deoxyribonucleic acid viruses. Similar results were found for influenza virus A2 Scotland/49 57, but not with vaccinia virus. In addition, the plaque titer of poliovirus for cells from normal individuals and patients with Down's syndrome was found to be the same (1). Thus, TS cell lines are less sensitive than TR cell lines to infection for some viruses but equally sensitive for others. The reasons for these differences is not known, but a possible explanation may lie in the differing ability of these viruses to replicate in human cells with the production of infective virus.

ACKNOWLEDGMENTS

The authors are indebted to C. H. Stuart-Harris and M. G. McEntegart, University of Sheffield, for their advice and criticism. We wish to thank P. Cockcroft, Doreen Coles, and G. Ellis for their excellent technical assistance.

This investigation was carried out with the financial assistance of the British Empire Cancer Campaign for Research.

LITERATURE CITED

1. Aaronson, S. A., and G. J. Todaro. 1968. SV40 T antigen induction and transformation in human fibroblast cell strains. Virology. 36:254–261.
2. Black, P. H. 1968. The oncogenic DNA viruses: a review of *in vitro* transformation studies. Annu. Rev. Microbiol. 22:391–426.
3. Fraumeni, J. E., and R. W. Miller. 1967. Epidemiology of human leukemia: recent observations. J. Nat. Cancer Inst. 38:593–605.
4. Huebner, R. J. 1967. Adenovirus-directed tumor and T antigens. *In* M. Pollard (ed.), Perspectives in virology, vol. 5. Academic Press Inc., New York.
5. Hyman, J. M. 1968. Culture of human fibroblasts for chromosome investigations. J. Med. Lab. Technol. 25:81–100.
6. Koprowski, H., J. A. Ponten, F. Jensen, R. G. Ravdin, P. Moorhead, and E. Saksela. 1962. Transformation of cultures of human tissue infected with simian virus SV40. J. Cell. Comp. Physiol. 59:281–292.
7. Miller, R. W., and G. J. Todaro. 1969. Viral transformation of cells from persons at high risk of cancer. Lancet 1:81–82.
8. Oxford, J. S., and C. W. Potter. 1969. Chick embryo lethal orphan (CELO) virus as a possible contaminant of egg-grown virus vaccines. J. Hyg. 67:41–47.
9. Oxford, J. S., and G. C. Schild. 1968. Immunofluorescent studies in the inhibition of influenza A and B viruses in mammalian cell culture by amines and ammonium compounds. J. Gen. Virol. 2:377–384.
10. Oxman, M. N., and P. H. Black. 1966. Inhibition of SV40 T antigen formation by interferon. Proc. Nat. Acad. Sci. U.S.A. 55:1133–1140.
11. Petek, M., B. Felloga, and R. Zoletto. 1963. Biological properties of CELO virus: stability to various agents, and electron microscopy. Avian Dis. 1:38–44.
12. Pope, J. H., and W. P. Rowe. 1964. Detection of specific antigen in SV40-transformed cells by immunofluorescence. J. Exp. Med. 120:124–128.
13. Potter, C. W., and J. S. Oxford. 1969. Specific tumour antigen induced by chick embryo lethal orphan (CELO) virus. J. Gen. Virol. 4:287–289.
14. Reed, L. J., and H. Muench. 1938. A simple method of estimating fifty per cent endpoints. Amer. J. Hyg. 27:493–497.
15. Sarma, P. S., R. J. Huebner, and W. T. Lane. 1965. Induction of tumours in hamsters with an avian adenovirus (CELO). Science (Washington) 149:1108–1109.
16. Shein, H. M., and J. F. Enders. 1962. Transformation induced by simian virus 40 in human renal cell cultures. 1. Morphology and growth characteristics. Proc. Nat. Acad. Sci. U.S.A. 48:1164–1172.
17. Todaro, G. J., H. Green, and M. R. Swift. 1966. Susceptibility of human diploid fibroblast strains to transformation by SV40 virus. Science (Washington) 153:1252–1254.
18. Todaro, G. J., and G. M. Martin. 1967. Increased susceptibility of Down's syndrome fibroblasts to transformation by SV40. Proc. Soc. Exp. Biol. Med. 124:1232–1236.

DETECTION OF SPECIFIC SURFACE ANTIGENS
BY COLONY INHIBITION IN CELLS TRANSFORMED
BY PAPOVAVIRUS SV40

by

Satvir S. Tevethia, Norman A. Crouch, Joseph L. Melnick and Fred Rapp

Transformation of mammalian cells by papovavirus SV40 results in the development of specific antigens at the cell surface. These antigens can be detected by the *in vivo* transplantation rejection test (Khera *et al.*, 1963; Defendi, 1963; Koch and Sabin, 1963; Habel and Eddy, 1963; Deichman and Kluchareva, 1964), by the *in vitro* immunofluorescence test (Tevethia *et al.*, 1965, 1968a; Kluchareva *et al.*, 1967; Girardi, 1967) and by the mixed hemadsorption test (Metzgar, 1968; Häyry and Defendi, 1968). Recently, the *in vitro* colony inhibition test has been applied to the demonstration of tumor immunity specific for polyoma virus (Hellström and Sjögren, 1966, 1967), adenovirus (Hellström and Sjögren, 1967), Shope papilloma virus (Hellström *et al.*, 1969a, b), Moloney sarcoma virus (Hellström and Hellström, 1969) and mouse mammary tumor virus (Heppner, 1969). The colony inhibition test has also been used to demonstrate immunity against autochthonous mouse tumors induced by methylcholanthrene (Hellström *et al.*, 1968b) and against human tumors (Hellström *et al.*, 1968a, c). Both cellular and humoral immunity have been demonstrated by the colony inhibition test.

Although the *in vitro* colony inhibition and immunofluorescence tests measure antigens at the surface of tumor cells, no evidence is available to show if both techniques measure the same antigen. This report describes the application of the *in vitro* colony inhibition test for the detection of SV40-specific antigens at the surface of SV40-transformed cells. A number of sera were tested both by the colony inhibition test and by the immunofluorescence test in an effort to obtain evidence that the two *in vitro* techniques measure the same or similar antigens.

Virus

SV40 was the Baylor reference strain described previously (Rapp *et al.*, 1965). The virus was grown in a continuous line of African green monkey kidney cell (CV-1) cultures maintained in Eagle's medium supplemented with 2% fetal calf serum, 100 units of penicillin and 100 μg of streptomycin per ml. At the time of maximum cytopathic effect, the virus was harvested by freezing and thawing the infected cultures three times in a dry-ice-alcohol bath and centrifuging the resulting suspension at low speed in the cold. The virus in the supernatant fluid was then treated with an equal amount of genetron. The genetron was removed by centrifugation at low speed in the cold. The treated virus was then centrifuged at $78,480 \times g$ for three hours using a No. 30 rotor in a Beckman Model L-2 Centrifuge. The pellet containing the virus was resuspended in Trisbuffered saline (TBS) and the resulting suspension was subjected to density gradient centrifugation in cesium chloride. The virus band at 1.33 g/cm³ was collected by puncturing the side of the tube with a tuberculin syringe, and dialyzed against TBS to remove the cesium chloride. The concentration of virus particles was determined by electron microscopy by the method of Smith and Melnick (1962).

Cell lines

The H-50 cells were derived from a hamster tumor induced by SV40 (Ashkenazi and Melnick, 1963). These cells synthesize the intranuclear SV40 tumor or T antigen (Rapp *et al.*, 1964) and contain SV40-specific surface (S) antigen(s) (Tevethia *et al.*, 1965; Tevethia and Rapp, 1965) and SV40 transplantation antigens (Khera *et al.*, 1963; Rapp *et al.*, 1966). The cells are free of

infectious virus (Melnick *et al.*, 1964). Normal hamster cells were derived from hamster embryos and these cells were devoid of any detectable SV40 markers.

Human cells transformed by SV40 were provided by Dr. David D. Porter (University of California at Los Angeles, USA) and contained SV40 T and transplantation antigen. Marmoset testicle cells were transformed by defective SV40; they contained SV40 T and transplantation antigens, but were free of infectious virus (Rapp and Layne, unpublished results). Normal marmoset testicle cells were also used as controls.

Antisera

Details for the preparation of antisera in hamsters are presented in Table I. The antisera in group A reacting against SV40-specific surface antigen(s) were prepared by inoculating hamsters subcutaneously with one injection of purified SV40. The virus dose consisted of 1×10^{11} physical virus particles. The hamsters were bled 40 days after the virus inoculation; the sera were collected and then stored at $-20°$ C until tested. It had previously been demonstrated that hamsters develop antibody to S antigens upon virus inoculation (Tevethia *et al.*, 1968a; Häyry and Defendi, 1968).

The sera in group B were prepared by immunizing hamsters with human cells transformed by SV40. The cells growing in 16-oz bottles were removed from the glass by trypsinization, washed three times with TBS and resuspended in TBS. Each hamster received six weekly intraperitoneal injections of 1×10^7 cells. The animals were bled one week after the last injection and the sera collected and stored at $-20°$ C.

The sera in group C were prepared in hamsters by means of marmoset cells transformed by

TABLE I

PREPARATION OF ANTISERUM IN HAMSTERS USED FOR THE TESTS

Serum group	Antigen	No. of inoculations	Amount per inoculation	Route
A	SV40, purified	1	1×10^{11} p.p. [1]	Subcutaneous
B	SV40-transformed human cells	6	1×10^7 cells	Intraperitoneal
C	SV40-transformed marmoset cells	6	1×10^7 cells	Intraperitoneal
D	Normal marmoset cells	6	1×10^7 cells	Intraperitoneal

[1] p.p. — physical particles.

defective SV40 in a manner similar to the preparation of antisera against SV40-transformed human cells. The sera in group D were prepared in hamsters against normal marmoset cells by the same procedure. All the sera were inactivated at 56° C for 30 minutes.

Immunofluorescence test

The indirect immunofluorescence tests for the detection of S antibody were carried out according to the method described by Möller (1961) and later modified (Tevethia *et al.*, 1968*a*). Briefly, the cells growing in tissue culture were brought into suspension with trypsin, washed once with growth medium containing 10 % fetal calf serum, and three times with TBS. After the final wash, 1×10^6 cells were reacted with the test serum. Following incubation for one hour at 37° C, the cells were washed three times with TBS and reacted with anti-hamster γ-globulin baboon γ-globulin conjugated with fluorescein isothiocyanate. After further incubation for 30 min at 37° C in the dark, the cells were washed three times, drained, suspended in buffered glycerol and examined in a Zeiss fluorescence microscope. Only the cells showing a bright green fluorescence in the form of a ring around the cell were counted as positive. Transformed as well as non-transformed cells were tested. The results of the immunofluorescence tests were expressed as fluorescence index (number of H-50 cells negative with normal hamster serum minus the number of H-50 cells negative with the test serum divided by the former figure). A serum was considered positive only if it had a fluorescence index of 0.3 or greater.

Colony inhibition test

The procedure of the colony inhibition test was only slightly modified from that described by Hellström and Sjögren (1965). Cells growing in 16-oz bottles in monolayer were trypsinized, washed and resuspended in Eagle's medium with 20 % fetal calf serum. The cells were then incubated for one hour at 37° C in Eagle's medium with 40 % fetal calf serum, after which the cells were centrifuged and diluted in the Eagle's medium to a concentration of 1×10^4 cells per ml. Of the diluted cell suspension, 0.1 ml (1×10^3 cells) was transferred to a 13×100 mm plastic tube fitted with a screw cap, and 0.1 ml of heat-inactivated normal or test serum was added to each tube. The cell-serum mixture was then

incubated at 37° C for 30 min, after which 0.4 ml of 1:5 diluted guinea-pig complement was added. After a further incubation for 45 min at 37° C, the 1.9 ml of medium was added to each tube and 0.5 ml of the suspension, containing 200 cells, was plated onto a 60 mm plastic Petri dish. Four plates were used for each serum sample. After addition of 4 ml of Eagle's medium supplemented with 20 % fetal calf serum to each plate, the plates were incubated at 37° C in a CO_2 atmosphere for six days at which time the fluid from the plates was drained off and the resulting colonies formed by the single cells were stained with crystal violet and counted. The inhibition of colony formation by the test sera was based on a comparison with the normal hamster sera. Experiments were also conducted in which heat-inactivated guinea-pig complement was substituted for the active complement.

RESULTS

The results of the *in vitro* colony inhibition test and its comparison with the immunofluorescence test are shown in Tables II to VII. Table II shows the results of colony inhibition and immunofluorescence tests with sera from hamsters immunized with purified SV40. The reaction of the normal hamster serum with the SV40-transformed hamster cells resulted in the formation of an average of 22 colonies. Of the eight immune sera tested, four inhibited colony formation by the SV40-transformed cells. The inhibition by the four sera ranged from 46 to 64 % when compared to the normal hamster serum. The immune sera from SV40-immunized hamsters, however, failed to inhibit the colony formation of non-transformed hamster cells. When tested by the immunofluorescence test, four of the eight sera also reacted positively with the SV40-transformed cells. The fluorescence indices of the four positive sera were 0.58, 0.58, 0.79 and 0.79. Three of the sera (282R, 281, 279L) reacted in both the tests. All sera reacted negatively in the immunofluorescence test with the non-transformed cells.

The results of the colony inhibition and the immunofluorescence tests with sera from hamsters prepared by inoculation of SV40-transformed human cells are shown in Table III. Seven of the eight sera reacted positively in the colony inhibition test. The inhibition ranged from 59 to 100 %. Two of the eight sera also inhibited the non-transformed hamster cells in the colony

TABLE II

IMMUNOFLUORESCENCE AND COLONY-INHIBITION TESTS WITH SERA FROM HAMSTERS
IMMUNIZED WITH PURIFIED SV40

Serum No.	SV40-transformed hamster cells [1]			Non-transformed hamster cells [1]		
	Fluorescence index	Average colonies per plate [2]±SD [3]	Percentage inhibition	Fluorescence index	Average colonies per plate [2]±SD [3]	Percentage inhibition
Normal sera	0.00	22±3.5	—	0.00	30±6.0	—
280RL	0.00	24±3.0	0	0.00	34±2.5	0
279-	0.00	33±5.4	0	0.00	34±3.2	0
279R	0.00	22±3.9	0	0.00	32±3.0	0
282R	0.79	12±4.1	46	0.00	37±5.4	0
281	0.79	9±1.9	59	0.00	32±7.4	0
279L	0.58	12±3.7	46	0.00	32±3.9	0
281R	0.58	24±3.0	0	0.00	30±2.3	0
282-	0.16	8±2.1	64	0.00	26±5.2	13

[1] The number of cells plated per Petri dish was 200.
[2] Average of four plates.
[3] SD, Standard deviation.

TABLE III

IMMUNOFLUORESCENCE AND COLONY-INHIBITION TESTS WITH SERA FROM HAMSTERS
IMMUNIZED WITH SV40-TRANSFORMED HUMAN CELLS

Serum No.	SV40-transformed hamster cells [1]			Non-transformed hamster cells [1]		
	Fluorescence index	Average colonies per plate [2]±SD [3]	Percentage inhibition	Fluorescence index	Average colonies per plate [2]±SD [3]	Percentage inhibition
Normal	0.00	22±3.2	—	0.00	30±6.0	—
X-69-1-1	0.10	20±2.9	9	0.01	NT [3]	—
X-69-1-2	0.89	9±1.8	59	0.01	30±6.7	0
X-69-1-3	1.00	0	100	0.09	10±3.1	67
X-69-1-4	1.00	3±1.6	86	0.01	5±2.1	83
X-69-1-5	1.00	5±1.5	77	0.01	35±8.4	0
X-69-1-6	1.00	3±1.1	86	0.01	32±5.9	0
X-69-1-7	0.57	6±1.1	73	0.01	29±2.8	3
X-69-1-8	0.57	2±1.3	91	0.01	NT [3]	—

[1] 200 cells were plated out per Petri dish.
[2] Average of four plates.
[3] SD — Standard deviation; NT — not tested.

inhibition test. Seven of the eight sera also reacted in the immunofluorescence test with the SV40-transformed cells; none of the seven sera reacted with the non-transformed cells by the immunofluorescence test. The same seven sera reacted in both tests.

Table IV shows the dependence of the inhibition of colony formation by the immune sera on the presence of active complement. The data showing the number of colonies formed after reaction with normal and immune serum in the presence of active guinea-pig complement are taken from Table III for comparison with the data obtained in the presence of inactivated complement. Reaction of the SV40-transformed cells with normal hamster serum resulted in the formation of an average of 22 colonies in the presence of inactivated complement. The same number was obtained in the presence of active complement and there was no inhibition of colony formation by the normal serum. The immune sera inhibited the transformed cells only in the

TABLE IV

REQUIREMENT OF ACTIVE COMPLEMENT FOR THE INHIBITION OF COLONY FORMATION
OF SV40-TRANSFORMED HAMSTER CELLS BY THE IMMUNE SERA

Serum No.	Average colonies per plate [1] ±SD [2]		Percentage inhibition based on inactivated complement control plus test serum	Percentage inhibition based on normal serum control plus active complement
	Inactivated guinea-pig complement [3]	Active guinea-pig complement [4]		
Normal serum	22±3.5	22±3.2	0	—
X-69-1-3	31 [5]	0	100	100
X-69-1-4	23±1.3	3±1.6	87	86
X-69-1-5	22±3.6	5±1.5	77	77
X-69-1-6	20±0.7	3±1.1	85	86
X-69-1-7	21±2.6	6±1.1	71	73
X-69-1-8	20±1.9	2±1.3	90	91

[1] Average of four Petri dishes; 200 cells were plated out per Petri dish.
[2] SD — standard deviation.
[3] Guinea-pig complement was heat inactivated at 56° C for 30 minutes.
[4] These data are taken from Table III for comparison with the colonies obtained in the presence of inactivated complement.
[5] Count of only one Petri dish.

TABLE V

IMMUNOFLUORESCENCE AND COLONY INHIBITION TESTS WITH SERA FROM HAMSTERS
IMMUNIZED WITH SV40-TRANSFORMED MARMOSET CELLS

Serum No.	SV40-transformed hamster cells [1]			Non-transformed hamster cells [2]		
	Fluorescence index	Average colonies per plate [3]±SD [4]	Percentage inhibition	Fluorescence index	Average colonies per plate [3]±SD [4]	Percentage inhibition
Normal	0.00	105±10.3	—	0.00	147±17.5	—
133R	0.00	100±4.2	5	NT [4]	NT [4]	—
133L	0.00	112±10.5	0	NT [4]	NT [4]	—
133RL	NT [4]	104±8.5	0	NT [4]	NT [4]	—
133	0.49	55±13.8	47	0.00	175±27.0	0
132	0.80	32±4.1	69	0.00	113±17.5	23
132RL	0.49	20±1.9	81	0.00	170±38.5	0

[1] 250 cells were plated out per Petri dish.
[2] 1,000 cells were plated out per Petri dish.
[3] Average of four plates.
[4] SD — Standard deviation; NT — not tested.

presence of active complement. The percentage inhibition of the transformed cells by the immune sera is the same when calculated either on the basis of the number of colonies obtained in the presence of test serum plus inactivated complement, or on the basis of the colonies obtained in the presence of normal serum and active complement. This indicates the specific immunological nature of the colony inhibition test.

Table V shows the results of colony inhibition and immunofluorescence tests with sera from hamsters prepared against SV40-transformed marmoset cells. Of the six sera tested, three reacted positively with SV40-transformed cells in the colony inhibition and the immunofluorescence tests. None of them reacted significantly with non-transformed cells.

The nature and specificity of the colony inhibition test were further tested by reacting sera from hamsters prepared against normal marmoset cells with the SV40-transformed hamster cells. The results presented in Table VI show that none

TABLE VI

COLONY-INHIBITION TESTS WITH SERA FROM HAMSTERS IMMUNIZED
WITH NORMAL MARMOSET CELLS

Serum No.	SV40-transformed hamster cells [1]		
	Fluorescence index	Average colonies per plate [2] +SD [3]	Percentage inhibition
Normal	0.00	105±10.3	—
130-	0.00	104±13.5	0
130RL	0.00	117±17.6	0
131R	0.00	97±4.9	7
131L	0.00	77±6.4	26
131-	0.00	84±3.8	19

[1] 250 cells were plated out per Petri dish.
[2] Average of four plates.
[3] SD — Standard deviation.

TABLE VII

COMPARISON OF COLONY INHIBITION AND IMMUNOFLUORESCENCE TESTS FOR THE DETECTION
OF SPECIFIC ANTIGENS AT THE SURFACE OF SV40-TRANSFORMED CELLS

" S " antibody against	Total sera tested	Sera positive by CI [1] or IF [1]	Sera positive by CI [1]	Sera positive by IF [1]	Sera positive by CI [1] and IF [1]
Purified SV40	8	5	4	4	3
SV40-transformed human cells	8	7	5	7	5
SV40-transformed marmoset cells	6	3	3	3	3
Total	22	15	12	14	11
Percentage positive	—	70	54	64	50

[1] CI = Colony inhibition test; IF = immunofluorescence test.

of the five sera tested inhibited significantly the colony formation of SV40-transformed hamster cells.

The results of the comparison of the colony inhibition test with the immunofluorescence test are summarized in Table VII. Four sera prepared against purified SV40 were positive in the colony inhibition test and the same number were positive in the immunofluorescence test. One reacted only by CI and three of the sera reacted in both the tests. Of eight sera prepared against SV40-transformed human cells, five reacted specifically in the CI test whereas seven reacted specifically in the IF test. Five sera reacted in both the tests. Of the six sera prepared against SV40-transformed marmoset cells, three reacted positively in both the tests. Of the total of 22 sera tested, 12 reacted positively in the colony inhibition test whereas

14 were positive in the immunofluorescence test Eleven of the sera reacted in both the tests. It is thus apparent that a high correlation exists between the colony inhibition and the immunofluorescence tests.

DISCUSSION

The present findings indicate that the *in vitro* colony inhibition test can be used to demonstrate specific antigens at the surface of SV40-transformed cells. In addition to specific antiserum, the colony inhibition reaction requires the presence of active complement. These findings extend the original observation of Hellström and Sjögren (1965, 1967) who used this test to demonstrate specific antigens at the surface of cells transformed by polyoma and adenovirus type 12.

Tumor-specific antigens at the cell surface have also been demonstrated by immunofluorescence in virus-induced tumors (Tevethia et al., 1965, 1968a; Kluchareva et al., 1967; Girardi, 1967; Irlin, 1967; Malmgren et al., 1968; Klein and Klein, 1964), in chemical carcinogen-induced tumors (Möller, 1964; Lejneva et al., 1965) and in Burkitt lymphoma cells (Klein et al., 1966). The evidence that the immunofluorescence technique is detecting transplantation antigens is, however, circumstantial. The colony inhibition test is believed to detect transplantation antigens. This is based on the assumption that the inhibition reaction with either lymphocytes or immune sera represents more closely the in vivo reaction of the immune host against the target tumor cells because the reaction measured in vivo and by the colony inhibition test results, in both cases, in death (inhibition) of the neoplastic cells. The results obtained in this study strongly suggest that the in vitro colony inhibition and the immunofluorescence tests detect the same antigen. Previous results (Tevethia et al., 1968a) have demonstrated that some of the SV40-transformed cells which lacked T antigen but contained S antigen detectable by the immunofluorescence technique, failed to be rejected by the SV40-immunized animals. This discrepancy between the immunofluorescence test and the in vivo transplant-rejection test may perhaps be explained by the assumption that the immunofluorescence test is more sensitive than the in vivo rejection test and that the T⁻S⁺ cells contain smaller amounts of transplantation antigens. It has been suggested (Diamandopoulos et al., 1968; Levin et al., 1969) that the S antigens detected at the surface of SV40-transformed cells are the result of derepression of the host cell genome by SV40. This possibility seems unlikely since antibody prepared in hamsters against SV40-transformed human and marmoset cells reacted specifically in immunofluorescence and colony inhibition tests with the SV40-transformed hamster cells. This common antigenicity of the specific surface antigens of the hamster, human and simian cells transformed by SV40 as demonstrated by the in vitro techniques correlates well with the common antigenicity demonstrated by the in vivo transplantation rejection test (Girardi, 1965; Jensen and Defendi, 1968). The common antigenicity of specific surface antigens has also been demonstrated between polyoma-virus-transformed hamster and mouse

cells by means of the in vivo rejection and in vitro colony inhibition tests (Hellström and Sjögren, 1966).

The ability of the immune sera to inhibit the SV40-transformed cells indicates that the humoral antibody may play some role in the rejection of the tumor cells by the immunized animals. Coggin and Ambrose (1969) have demonstrated that the SV40-immunized animals can successfully check the growth of virus-free transformed cells contained in a Millipore diffusion chamber implanted in the peritoneal cavity of the immune host. Girardi (1967) has demonstrated that the humoral antibodies from SV40-immunized hamsters which react positively in the immunofluorescence test can enhance the SV40-tumor cell transplants in the immune hamsters which had previously rejected a tumor cell transplant.

However, the tumor-inhibiting and tumor-enhancing role of humoral antibodies from immune hamsters may be explained by postulating that the inhibition of the tumor cells is mediated by 7Sγ2 immunoglobulin which has the ability to fix complement whereas enhancement is mediated by 7Sγ1 immunoglobulin. The presence of two types of 7S immunoglobulin, γ1 and γ2, in the hamster sera has been documented (Tevethia, 1967; Fugmann and Sigel, 1967; Coe, 1968). Recently, Hellström and Hellström (1969), using in vitro colony inhibition, have demonstrated that the sera from mice bearing Moloney sarcomas protect the sarcoma cells against the inhibitory action of immune lymphocytes whereas the sera from animals showing spontaneous regression do not have this protective effect. Whether the same situation exists in vivo is not known at the present time. Studies are in progress to investigate the type of immunoglobulins reacting in the colony inhibition and immunofluorescence tests and in the immunological enhancement of tumor transplants.

ACKNOWLEDGEMENTS

Supported in part by Public Health Service research grant CA 04600 and contract PH 43-68-678 from the National Cancer Institute, and training grant 2T1 AI-74 from the National Institute of Allergy and Infectious Diseases, National Institutes of Health. Miss Virginia L. McMillan provided excellent technical assistance and Mrs. Liane Jordan carried out the electron microscopy.

ASHKENAZI, A., and MELNICK, J. L., Tumorigenicity of simian papovavirus SV40 and of virus-transformed cells. *J. nat. Cancer Inst.*, **30**, 1227-1265 (1963).

COE, J. E., The immune response in the hamster. I. Definition of two 7S globulin classes: 7Sγ1 and 7Sγ2. *J. Immunol.*, **100**, 507-515 (1968).

COGGIN, J. H., JR., and AMBROSE, K. R., A rapid *in vivo* assay for SV40 tumor immunity in hamsters. *Proc. Soc. exp. Biol. (N.Y.)*, **130**, 246-252 (1969).

DEFENDI, V., Effects of SV40-virus immunization on growth of transplantable SV40 and polyoma-virus tumors in hamsters. *Proc. Soc. exp. Biol. (N.Y.)*, **113**, 12-16 (1963).

DEICHMAN, G. K., and KLUCHAREVA, T. E., Immunological determinants of oncogenesis in hamsters infected with SV40 virus. *Virology*, **24**, 131-137 (1964).

DIAMANDOPOULOS, G. Th., TEVETHIA, S. S., RAPP, F., and ENDERS, J. F., Development of S and T antigens and oncogenicity in hamster embryonic cell lines exposed to SV40. *Virology*, **34**, 331-336 (1968).

FUGMANN, R. A., and SIGEL, M. M., Nature of hamster complement-fixing antibody to adenovirus 12 tumor antigen. *J. Virol.*, **1**, 678-683 (1967).

GIRARDI, A. J., Prevention of SV40 virus oncogenesis in hamsters. I. Tumor resistance induced by human cells transformed by SV40. *Proc. nat. Acad. Sci. (Wash.)*, **54**, 445-451 (1965).

GIRARDI, A. J., Tumor resistance and tumor enhancement with SV40 virus-induced tumors. *In:* Cottier, H., Odartchenko, N., Schindler, R., and Congdon, C. C. (ed.) *Germinal centers in immune responses*, pp. 422-427, Springer-Verlag, New York (1967).

HABEL, K., and EDDY, B. E., Specificity of resistance to tumor challenge of polyoma and SV40 virus-immune hamsters. *Proc. Soc. exp. Biol. (N.Y.)*, **113**, 1-4 (1963).

HÄYRY, P., and DEFENDI, V., Use of mixed hemagglutination technique in detection of virus-induced antigen(s) on SV40-transformed cell surface. *Virology*, **36**, 317-321 (1968).

HELLSTRÖM, I., EVANS, C. A., and HELLSTRÖM, K. E., Cellular immunity and its serum-mediated inhibition in Shope-virus-induced papillomas. *Int. J. Cancer*, **4**, 601-607 (1969a).

HELLSTRÖM, I., and HELLSTRÖM, K. E., Studies on cellular immunity and its serum-mediated inhibition in Moloney-virus-induced mouse sarcomas. *Int. J. Cancer*, **4**, 587-598 (1969).

HELLSTRÖM, I., HELLSTRÖM, K. E., EVANS, C. A., HEPPNER, G. H., PIERCE, G. E., and YANG, J. P. S., Serum mediated protection of neoplastic cells from inhibition of lymphocytes immune to their tumor specific antigens. *Proc. nat. Acad. Sci. (Wash.)*, **62**, 362-369 (1969b).

HELLSTRÖM, I., HELLSTRÖM, K. E., and PIERCE, G. E., *In vitro* studies of immune reactions against autochthonous and syngeneic mouse tumors induced by methylcholanthrene and plastic discs. *Int. J. Cancer*, **3**, 467-482 (1968a).

HELLSTRÖM, I., HELLSTRÖM, K. E., PIERCE, G. E., and BILL, A. H., Demonstration of cell-bound and humoral immunity against neuroblastoma cells. *Proc. nat. Acad. Sci. (Wash.)*, **60**, 1231-1238 (1968b).

HELLSTRÖM, I., HELLSTRÖM, K. E., PIERCE, G. E., and YANG, J. P. S., Cellular and humoral immunity to different types of human neoplasms. *Nature (Lond.)*, **220**, 1352-1354 (1968c).

HELLSTRÖM, I., and SJÖGREN, H. O., Demonstration of H-2 isoantigens and polyoma specific tumor antigens by measuring colony formation *in vitro*. *Exp. Cell Res.*, **40**, 212-215 (1965).

HELLSTRÖM, I., and SJÖGREN, H. O., Demonstration of common specific antigen(s) in mouse and hamster polyoma tumors. *Int. J. Cancer*, **1**, 481-489 (1966).

HELLSTRÖM, I., and SJÖGREN, H. O., *In vitro* demonstration of humoral and cell-bound immunity against common specific transplantation antigen(s) of adenovirus 12-induced mouse and hamster tumors. *J. exp. Med.*, **125**, 1105-1118 (1967).

HEPPNER, G. H., Studies on serum-mediated inhibition of cellular immunity to spontaneous mouse mammary tumors. *Int. J. Cancer*, **4**, 608-615 (1969).

IRLIN, I. S., Immunofluorescent demonstration of a specific surface antigen in cells infected or transformed by polyoma virus. *Virology*, **32**, 725-728 (1967).

JENSEN, F., and DEFENDI, V., Transformation of African green monkey kidney cells by irradiated adenovirus 7-simian virus 40 hybrid. *J. Virol.*, **2**, 173-177 (1968).

KHERA, K. S., ASHKENAZI, A., RAPP, F., and MELNICK, J. L., Immunity in hamsters to cells transformed *in vitro* and *in vivo* by SV40. Tests for antigenic relationship among the papovaviruses. *J. Immunol.*, **91**, 604-613 (1963).

KLEIN, E., and KLEIN, G., Antigenic properties of lymphomas induced by the Moloney agent. *J. nat. Cancer Inst.*, **32**, 547-568 (1964).

KLEIN, G., CLIFFORD, P., KLEIN, E., and STJERNSWÄRD, J., Search for tumor-specific immune reactions in Burkitt lymphoma patients by the membrane immunofluorescence reaction. *Proc. nat. Acad. Sci. (Wash.)*, **55**, 1628-1635 (1966).

KLUCHAREVA, T. E., SHACKANINA, K. L., BELOVA, S., CHIBISOVA, V., and DEICHMAN, G. I., Use of immunofluorescence for detection of specific membrane antigens in simian virus 40-infected nontransformed cells. *J. nat. Cancer Inst.*, **39**, 825-832 (1967).

KOCH, M. A., and SABIN, A. B., Specificity of virus-induced resistance to transplantation of polyoma and SV-40 tumors in adult hamsters. *Proc. Soc. exp. Biol. (N.Y.)*, **113**, 4-12 (1963).

LEJNEVA, O. M., ZILBER, L. A., and ILULEVA, E. S., Humoral antibodies to methylcholanthrene sarcomata detected by a fluorescent technique. *Nature (Lond.)*, **206**, 1163-1164 (1965).

LEVIN, M. J., OXMAN, M. N., DIAMANDOPOULOS, G. Th., LEVINE, A. S., HENRY, P. H., and ENDERS, J. F., Virus-specific nucleic acids in SV40-exposed hamster embryo cell lines: Correlation with S and T antigens. *Proc. nat. Acad. Sci. (Wash.)*, **62**, 589-596 (1969).

MALMGREN, R. A., TAKEMOTO, K. K., and CARNEY, P. G., Immunofluorescent studies of mouse

and hamster cell surface antigens induced by polyoma virus. *J. nat. Cancer Inst.*, **40**, 263-268 (1968).

MELNICK, J. L., KHERA, K. S., and RAPP, F., Papovavirus SV40: Failure to isolate infectious virus from transformed hamster cells synthesizing SV40-induced antigens. *Virology*, **23**, 430-432 (1964).

METZGAR, R. S., and OLEINICK, S. R., The study of normal and malignant cell antigens by mixed agglutination. *Cancer Res.*, **28**, 1366-1371 (1968).

MÖLLER, G., Demonstration of mouse isoantigens at the cellular level by the fluorescent antibody technique. *J. exp. Med.*, **114**, 415-434 (1961).

MÖLLER, G., Effect on tumor growth in syngeneic recipients of antibodies against tumor-specific antigens in methylcholanthrene-induced mouse sarcomas. *Nature (Lond.)*, **204**, 846-847 (1964).

RAPP, F., BUTEL, J. S., FELDMAN, L. A., KITAHARA, T., and MELNICK, J. L., Differential effects of inhibitors on the steps leading to the formation of SV40 tumor and virus antigens. *J. exp. Med.*, **121**, 935-944 (1965).

RAPP, F., BUTEL, J. S., and MELNICK, J. L., Virus-induced intranuclear antigen in cells transformed by papovavirus SV40. *Proc. Soc. exp. Biol. (N.Y.)*, **116**, 1131-1135 (1964).

RAPP, F., TEVETHIA, S. S., and MELNICK, J. L., Papovavirus SV40 transplantation immunity conferred by an adenovirus SV40 hybrid. *J. nat. Cancer Inst.*, **36**, 703-708 (1966).

SMITH, K. O., and MELNICK, J. L., A method for staining virus particles and identifying the nucleic acid type in the electron microscope. *Virology*, **17**, 480-490 (1962).

TEVETHIA, S. S., Characterization of hamster antibody reacting with papovavirus SV40 tumor antigen. *J. Immunol.*, **98**, 1257-1264 (1967).

TEVETHIA, S. S., COUVILLON, L. A., and RAPP, F., Development in hamsters of antibodies against surface antigens present in cells transformed by papovavirus SV40. *J. Immunol.*, **100**, 358-362 (1968a).

TEVETHIA, S. S., DIAMANDOPOULOS, G. Th., RAPP, F., and ENDERS, J. F., Lack of relationship between virus-specific surface and transplantation antigens in hamster cells transformed by simian papovavirus SV40. *J. Immunol.*, **101**, 1192-1198 (1968b).

TEVETHIA, S. S., KATZ, M., and RAPP, F., New surface antigen in cells transformed by simian papova virus SV40. *Proc. Soc. exp. Biol. (N.Y.)*, **119**, 896-901 (1965).

TEVETHIA, S. S., and RAPP, F., Demonstration of new surface antigens in cells transformed by papovavirus SV40 by cytotoxic tests. *Proc. Soc. exp. Biol. (N.Y.)*, **120**, 455-458 (1965).

DETECTION OF TUMOR-SPECIFIC CELL SURFACE ANTIGEN
OF SIMIAN VIRUS 40-INDUCED TUMORS
BY THE ISOTOPIC ANTIGLOBULIN TECHNIQUE

by

Chou-Chik TING and Ronald B. HERBERMAN

Tumor-specific cell surface antigens of Papova-virus-induced tumors have been demonstrated by various *in vitro* assays; colony inhibition test (Hellström, 1965), immunofluorescent technique (Tevethia *et al.*, 1965; Irlin, 1967; Malmgren *et al.*, 1968), mixed hemagglutination test (Häyry and Defendi, 1970), cytotoxicity test (Smith *et al.*, 1970) and isotopic antiglobulin technique (Ting and Herberman, 1970). The nature of the surface antigens detected by these methods and their relationship to each other, especially their relationship to TSTA, is not well understood. The isotopic antiglobulin technique (IAT) is a sensitive and quantitative assay for cell surface antigens (Sparks *et al.*, 1969; Ting and Herberman, 1970). It has been successfully utilized to detect the polyoma tumor-specific cell surface and antigen (Ting and Herberman, 1970). In the present study, this technique has been extended to detect SV40 tumor-specific cell surface antigen, and the antigenic content of various SV40-transformed cell lines has been determined. Quantitative analysis of the antigens provided better confirmation of their specificity. The quantitative relationship of the surface antigen to TSTA and T antigen has also been studied.

MATERIAL AND METHODS

Mice

Male and female A/LN mice were obtained from the Animal Production Branch, Division of Research Services, National Institutes of Health, Bethesda, Md., USA. Mice of the same age were used in each experiment.

The SV-A/LN cells were very immunogenic in syngeneic A/LN mice; tumors could only be produced in irradiated or thymectomized mice (Takemoto *et al.*, 1968). This strain was therefore very suitable for the study of the immune response to tumor antigen, since large numbers of tumor cells could be used for immunization without the production of progressively growing tumors. The SV40 tumors were produced by subcutaneous inoculation of SV-A/LN tissue culture cells into A/LN mice which had received 350-400 R irradiation. Three to 4 weeks after inoculation, the resultant tumors were 0.5-1.5 cm in diameter. They were removed, minced finely and suspended in normal saline. The tumor cells were given to adult (non-irradiated) A/LN mice by trocar inoculation. The dosage of the tumor cells was divided into three categories: a) High dose (tumor brei from two 1.5 cm diameter tumors given to 10 mice); b) moderate dose (one 1.5 cm diameter tumor given to 10 mice); c) low dose (one 0.5 cm diameter tumor given to 10 mice). The mice were immunized with 1 to 4 such doses at weekly intervals. These mice were bled from the retro-orbital sinuses at various times during and after immunization; sera within the same experimental group were pooled and stored at −20° C until testing. Pooled normal serum was obtained in the same manner from non-immunized mice of the same age.

Test cells

Tissue culture cells were used in the experiments. They were grown as monolayers in 8-oz plastic tissue culture flasks (Falcon Plastics, Los Angeles, Calif., USA) with Eagle's basal medium containing 10% fetal bovine serum (FBS, Grand Island Biological Co., Grand Island, N.Y., USA). They were harvested by trypsinization with 0.2% crystalline trypsin in Tris-buffered saline and were transferred to spinner culture flasks (Bellco Glass, Inc., Vineland, New Jersey, USA) with Eagle's minimum essential medium (spinner) containing 10% FBS for at least 20-24 h before testing.

1) SV-A/LN: originated from inbred A/LN mouse embryo cells, transformed by SV40

93

(Takemoto et al., 1968).

2) A/LN: originated from inbred A/LN mouse embryo cells (Takemoto et al., 1968).

3) Py-A/LN: originated from inbred A/LN mouse embryo cells, transformed by polyoma virus (obtained from Dr. K. K. Takemoto).

4) mKS-A: originated from inbred BALB/c mouse kidney cells, transformed by SV40 (Kit et al., 1969).

5) 1807: originated from hamster embryo cells, transformed after exposure to SV40. These were the cells designated as T⁻S⁺ by Tevethia et al., (Levin et al., 1969).

6) 1808: originated from hamster embryo cells, transformed by SV40. This was one of the T⁺S cell lines used in studies of Tevethia et al. (Levin et al., 1969).

7) 1809: originated from hamster embryo cells, spontaneously transformed. This line was designated as T⁻S⁻ cells by Tevethia et al. (Levin et al., 1969).

8) 2952: originated from hamster embryo cells, transformed by SV40. This line was designated as T⁺S⁺ cells by Tevethia et al. (Levin et al., 1969 [1]).

9) PyT54: originated from hamster cells, transformed by polyoma virus (Takemoto et al., 1966).

Some characteristics of these cell lines are given in Table I.

Isotopic antiglobulin test (IAT)

Details of the technique have been described in a previous paper (Sparks et al., 1969). One tenth ml of test sera or normal serum at the same dilution was incubated with test cells in 10×75 mm test tubes at room temperature for 30 min. The cells were washed 5-7 times with barbital buffered saline (BBS) containing 10% FBS. A second incubation with 2 μl of ^{125}I-labelled anti-mouse gamma globulin (kindly provided by Dr. R. Asof-

---

[1] The hamster cell line 2952 was originally designated as clone P-10 by Enders and Diamandopoulos (1969).

TABLE I

Cell lines	SV40 T antigen	SV40 TSTA	Surface antigen (by Tevethia et al.)	Surface antigen by IAT [2]
SV-A/LN	+	+	NT	+
A/LN	−	NT	NT	−
Py-A/LN [1]	−	NT	NT	−
mKS-A	+	+	NT	+
1807	−	−	+	−
1808	+	+	+	+
1809	−	−	−	−
2952	+	+	+	+
PyT54 [1]	−	NT	NT	−

[1] Possessed polyoma T antigen.
[2] IAT: Isotopic antiglobulin technique.
NT = Not tested.

TABLE II

DIRECT TESTING WITH ANTISERUM (a.s.)
(No. 3187) AND NORMAL SERUM (n.s.) (No. 3189) at 1:64

Test cells	cpm of antiserum	cpm of normal serum	AR $\frac{\text{cpm a.s.}}{\text{cpm n.s.}}$
1807 [1]	3949	3454	1.1
1808 [1]	3713	2457	1.5
1809 [1]	3348	3699	0.9
2952 [1]	4543	2289	2.0
SV-A/LN [2]	8209	2662	3.1

[1] 2×10^5 cells were incubated with 0.1 ml of serum.
[2] 1×10^5 cells were incubated with 0.1 ml of serum.

sky, National Institutes of Allergy and Infectious Diseases) was done at 4° C for 15 min. The cells were again washed five times with BBS/10% FBS and transferred to plastic tubes to be counted in a gamma scintillation counter (Nuclear Chicago Corp., Des Plaines, Ill., USA). All tests were done in duplicate or triplicate.

Activity of the test sera was expressed as counts per minute (cpm) of ^{125}I-antiglobulin bound to the cells when a standard control serum was used in each experiment, or expressed as the absorption ratio (AR):

$$AR = \frac{^{125}\text{I counts from cells incubated with mouse antiserum} + {}^{125}\text{I-antiglobulin}}{^{125}\text{I counts from cells incubated with mouse normal serum} + {}^{125}\text{I-antiglobulin}}$$

A reaction was defined as positive when AR was equal to, or greater than, 2. For screening purposes, 0.1 ml of test sera or normal serum at 1:10 dilution was incubated with SV-A/LN, A/LN or Py-A/LN tissue culture cells. The test sera which only gave positive reactions with SV-A/LN cells were then tested at further dilutions to determine their titers. The antibody titer was defined as the highest dilution of serum giving an AR greater than 2.

Absorption of antiserum activity

Four tenths ml of antiserum at a dilution that still gave an AR greater than 2 were incubated with varying numbers of cells at 37° C for 1 h, with frequent mixing. The cell suspensions were then centrifuged at 2,000 × g for 15 min. The supernatant serum was carefully removed and then tested against SV-A/LN cells for residual activity, as described earlier. The cpm obtained with the absorbed antiserum was compared to the cpm obtained with the same dilution of normal serum, absorbed in the same manner.

Absorption of 50% of the antiserum activity was defined as the midpoint of the maximal and minimal cpm obtained with the absorbed antiserum. The minimal cpm that could be achieved was in the range of cpm of absorbed normal serum.

I. Direct testing

A. Screening of the immune sera. All the immune sera prepared by different schedules were tested against the syngeneic SV40-transformed cell line SV-A/LN and parent cell lines A/LN or polyoma virus transformed cell line Py-A/LN. The results obtained with SV-A/LN cells are shown in Figure 1. The ARs were from 1.0 to 3.5. The peak level was at 2-5 weeks after the last dose of immunizing tumor cells or after tumor regression. In tumor-bearing mice or during the course of immunization, little or no antibody activity was detectable. High antibody activity was present only in the sera of tumor-free mice, or after regression of the tumor. One high dose or two medium doses (Group I, IV) of tumor cells produced a good antibody response (Fig. 1). In the hyperimmunized mice (in Group I, the tumors persisted for 3-4 weeks; in Group VI, all mice received four high doses at weekly intervals) the antibody remained at a high level for a longer period of time. Those mice which received very high doses of tumor cells (Group V) became emaciated after immunization, which could be the cause of weak antibody response. The mice which only received one low dose (Group II) did not show evidence of any antibody production.

When these sera were tested against A/LN or Py-A/LN cells, the ARs obtained were from 0.8 to 1.6. None of the sera gave an AR greater than 2 with these cells. The reactions of these sera with only SV40-transformed cells demonstrated the SV40 specificity of the antisera.

After a number of sera had been screened, two (No. 3187 and No. 3193) were used for more extensive studies. The titers of these sera were greater than 1:512 (Fig. 2). Absorption experiments were then possible at these high dilutions of antisera.

B. Testing with hamster cells. Four cell lines: 1807, 1808, 1809 and 2952 were tested with antiserum No. 3187 and normal serum No. 3189 at 1:64 dilution. SV-A/LN cells were used as positive controls. The results are summarized in Table II. A positive reaction was only obtained with 2952 cells, with AR of 2. Negative reactions

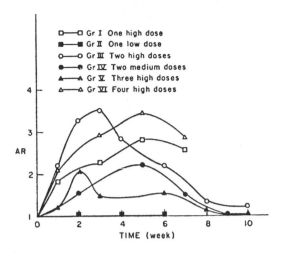

FIGURE 1

Kinetics of the antibody response to SV40 tumor-specific cell surface antigen obtained by immunization of the A/LN mice with various doses of syngeneic SV-A/LN tumors. The immune sera and normal sera were tested at 1:10 dilution with SV-A/LN cells. The activity of the immune sera was expressed as AR (absorption ratio).

were obtained with 1807 and 1809 cells. The reaction with 1808 was also negative, with an AR of 1.5.

II. Absorption experiments

Absorption experiments were performed to confirm the specificity of the reactions. The absorption assays were also used to determine the content of the surface antigens in various cell lines (Ting and Herberman, 1970), since quantitative analysis of the TSSA might provide important evidence as to its relationship to TSTA.

A. Confirmation of the specificity. Antiserum No. 3187 and normal serum No. 3189 at 1:300 were absorbed with SV-A/LN, A/LN and Py-A/LN cells. The results are summarized in Table III. The activity of the antiserum was only inhibited by absorption with SV-A/LN cells. The positive absorption by SV-A/LN could not be attributed to histocompatibility differences, since the parent cell line A/LN and Py-A/LN, which possessed the same histocompatibility antigens, did not remove the activity from the antiserum. In some instances, absorption with non-SV40 cells reduced the ^{125}I counts obtained with the antiserum, but the ARs did not decrease or even increase because ^{125}I counts were also reduced after absorption of the normal serum. This phenomenon was also seen in the polyoma system (Ting and Herberman, 1970). Only absorption with the SV-A/LN cells reduced both the ^{125}I cpm and AR. These findings confirmed that the reactions obtained with the antiserum were specific for SV40-transformed cells (Fig. 3).

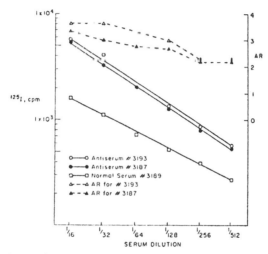

FIGURE 2

Reaction of two antisera and normal serum with SV-A/LN cells. ^{125}I cpm and AR obtained with various dilutions of each serum are shown.

B. Relationship of TSSA to TSTA and T antigen. Tevethia *et al.* (1968) have reported that there was a lack of relationship between TSSA (or " S " antigen), T antigen and TSTA, in SV40-induced tumors. Some of the cell lines used in their experiments were tested here; these were four hamster cell lines which had been classified as $T^{+}S^{+}$ cells (1808, 2952), $T^{-}S^{+}$ cells (1807) and $T^{-}S^{-}$ cells (1809) for SV40 surface antigen and T antigen, as assayed by immunofluorescent technique (Levin *et al.*, 1969). In addition to these cells, a BALB/c mouse cell line which was transformed by SV40 (mSK-A) was also used in the absorption experiments. These experiments were performed at 1:600 serum dilution. The results are summarized in Table IV. These experiments showed that the " T^-S^+ " cells (1807) as well as the " T^-S^- " cells (1809) did not have detectable TSSA. Only the " T^+S^+ " cells (1808, 2952) had a considerable amount of TSSA, but they differed from each other in quantity. The amount of TSSA per cell was 4-5 times more in 2952 cells than 1808 cells. An allogeneic SV40-transformed cell line mKS-A which possessed both TSTA and T antigen also had a considerable amount of TSSA, only slightly less than the SV-A/LN cells. It has been previously shown that only the " T^+S^+ " cells had a detectable amount of TSTA (Tevethia *et al.*, 1968). Thus, our data indicated a parallel expression of these three tumor-specific antigens—TSSA, TSTA and T antigen.

DISCUSSION

The IAT was successfully used to assay SV40 TSSA. Specific antisera could be produced by giving one or two large doses of SV-A/LN tumor cells. The antibody was usually not detectable or present in very low amounts during the course of immunization or in tumor-bearing mice. This suggested that the antibody might be absorbed *in vivo* by the tumor cells; it became detectable only when most of the tumor cells had been eradicated. This finding was reminiscent of our previous observation of early reduction of humoral antibody response by second set mouse skin allografts (Sparks *et al* 1970; Ting and Herberman, 1971). The peak of the antibody response was usually between 2 and 5 weeks after the last dose of immunization or after tumor regression. This pattern was also similar to the antibody response to polyoma tumor in syngeneic C3H/HeN mice (Ting and Herberman, 1970). It is difficult to comment on whether this pattern of antibody response generally applies to all DNA virus-induced tumors, since only two papova-virus-induced tumors have been studied. This relationship of antibody to tumor growth, however, is different from that observed with an RNA virus (Gross) induced tumor (Herberman *et al.*,

TABLE III

ABSORPTION OF ANTISERUM (a.s.) (No. 3187) AND NORMAL SERUM (n.s.) (No. 3189) at 1:300

Cells used for absorption	Number of cells used	cpm of antiserum	cpm of normal serum	AR cpm a.s. / cpm n.s.	Number of cells to absorb 50% activity [2]
		2216	872	2.5	
SV-A/LN	1.5×10^7	626	540	1.1	
	4.5×10^6	1348	840	1.6	4.6×10^6
	1.5×10^6	1972	690	2.5	
A/LN	2.6×10^7	1938	636	3.0	No absorption up to 2.6×10^7 cells
	7.8×10^6	2358	946	2.5	
	2.6×10^6	2028	810	2.6	
Py-A/LN	2.0×10^7	1826	648	2.8	No absorption up to 2.0×10^7 cells
	6.0×10^6	2322	700	3.3	
	2.0×10^6	2026	602	2.8	
PyT54 [1]	4×10^7	2057	786	2.7	No absorption up to 4×10^7 cells
	1.2×10^7	2026	716	2.8	
	4×10^6	2131	814	2.5	

[1] PyT54 cells were incubated with 0.2% trypsin for 10 min, washed twice with Eagle's basal medium, then suspended in BBS/10% FBS.
[2] 50% activity corresponds to 1350 cpm of [125]I.

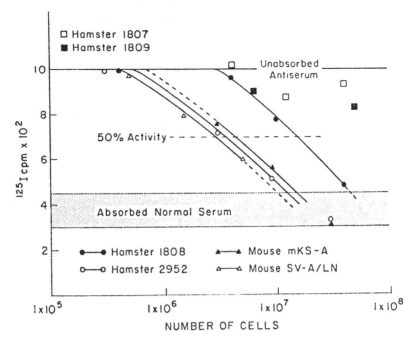

FIGURE 3

Antiserum (No. 3187) and normal serum (No. 3189) at 1:600 dilution were absorbed with various numbers of SV40-transformed cell lines and with non-SV40 cells. Absorbed and unabsorbed sera were then tested for residual activity with SV-A/LN cells. The range of ^{125}I cpm obtained with the absorbed normal serum is shown by the dotted area.

1971).

The nature of the TSSA detected by various *in vitro* assays is very controversial. Recently, questions have been raised regarding the specificity of these antigens and their relationship to other tumor antigens (Tevethia *et al.*, 1968). By using the IAT, SV40 TSSA was only found in the syngeneic, allogeneic or xenogeneic SV40-transformed cells. It was not detected in untransformed cells or in polyoma virus-transformed cells. Absorption experiments performed with trypsin-treated cells showed that non-SV40 cells did not become reactive, and that the SV40 transformed cells actually became somewhat less reactive (Table III and unpublished data). All of these data indicated that the TSSA of SV40 tumor cells detected in the present study was virus-

TABLE IV

ABSORPTION OF ANTISERUM (a.s.) (No. 3187) AND NORMAL SERUM (n.s.) (No. 3189) AT 1:600

Cells used for absorption	Number of cells used	cpm of antiserum	cpm of normal serum	AR cpm a.s. cpm n.s.	Number of cells to absorb 50% activity [1]
		1080	451	2.4	
1807	4×10^7	936	271	3.4	No absorption up to 4×10^7 cells
	1.2×10^7	874	315	2.8	
	4×10^6	1015	346	3.0	
1808	4×10^7	483	317	1.5	1.5×10^7 cells
	1.2×10^7	778	364	2.1	
	4×10^6	969	453	2.1	
	4×10^5	1019	421	2.4	
1809	5×10^7	838	227	3.7	No absorption up to 5×10^7
	5×10^6	897	355	2.5	
2952	3×10^7	336	243	1.4	3.4×10^6 cells
	9×10^6	519	265	1.9	
	3×10^6	718	321	2.2	
	3×10^5	993	437	2.2	
mKS-A	3×10^7	305	255	1.2	4.2×10^6 cells
	9×10^6	566	318	1.7	
	3×10^6	750	371	2.0	
SV-A/LN	5×10^6	605	400	1.5	2.7×10^6 cells
	1.5×10^6	789	345	2.2	
	5×10^5	972	386	2.4	

[1] 50% activity point corresponds to ^{125}I cpm of 700.

specific and did not appear to be a normal cellular antigen " uncovered " by viral transformation or by trypsin treatment.

The TSSA was only present in considerable amounts in T antigen-positive cells which also possessed TSTA, *i.e.* two mouse cell lines (SV-A/LN, mKS-A) and two hamster cell lines (1808, 2952). The " T^-S^+ " cells or " T^-S^- " cells did not have detectable amounts of TSSA. This parallel expression of TSSA and TSTA is consistent with the hypothesis that the TSSA detected by the IAT related to SV40 viral gene expression and was the same as TSTA. The absence of detectable amounts of specific viral RNA or viral DNA in the " T^-S^+ " cells was in support of this hypothesis (Levin *et al.*, 1969; Levine *et al.*, 1970). The surface antigen of the " $T^ S^+$ " cells, which had no TSTA, was not related to the viral genome and, thus, might not really be virus-specific.

The discrepancy between our findings and those of Tevethia *et al.* could be due to the following reasons: (a) Methods of antiserum preparation: to eliminate any undesirable antibody production to fetal bovine serum antigens or antigens related to trypsinization, tissue culture cells or preparations containing fetal bovine serum were not used for our immunization. Fresh tumor cells suspended in normal saline were used in all immunizations; (b) antiglobulin reagent: the potency and specificity of the antiglobulin reagent are critical factors for both the immunofluorescent test and IAT; (c) differences in assays: the IAT seems to be a more sensitive assay. Absorption experiments allow detection of smaller amounts of antigen. For instance, while only one of the two SV40-transformed hamster cell lines (2952, 1808) was positive by direct testing at 1:64 serum dilution (Table II), absorption experiments showed that both had SV40 TSSA. However, 2952 cells had more of this antigen (Table IV); (d) difference in antigen: the surface antigen of T^-S^+ cells might be a normal component of hamster cells but not of the mouse cells. The exposure to simian virus 40 might " uncover " or de-repress the synthesis of this antigen. Thus, it was present in both " T^-S^+ " or " T^+S^+ " hamster cells. Since the antisera used in the present study were produced in mice, they would not react with a species (hamster) specific antigen of " T⁻S⁺ " hamster cells.

Therefore, from the above observations, it can be concluded that the TSSA of SV40-transformed cells was virus-specific. It was only detected in the cells which also had both the SV40 T antigen and TSTA. The quantitative expressions of these three antigens were closely related and may be regulated by the activity of the viral genome incorporated into the transformed cells.

ACKNOWLEDGEMENT

We are very grateful to Dr. M. N. Oxman and Dr. G. Th. Diamandopoulos for supplying the hamster tissue culture cells. We thank Miss G. Shiu, Mr. W. Lyles and Mrs. H. Porter for their excellent technical assistance.

REFERENCES

ENDERS, J. F., and DIAMANDOPOULOS, G. Th., A study of variation and progression in oncogenicity in an SV40-transformed hamster heart cell line and its clones. *Proc. roy. Soc., Ser. B*, **171**, 431-443 (1969).

HÄYRY, P., and DEFENDI, V., Surface antigen(s) of SV40-transformed tumor cells. *Virology*, **41**, 22-29 (1970).

HELLSTRÖM, I., Distinction between the effect of antiviral and anticellular polyoma antibodies on polyoma tumor cells. *Nature (Lond.)*, **208**, 652-653 (1965).

HERBERMAN, R. B., and OREN, M. E., Immune response to Gross virus-induced lymphoma. I. Kinetics of cytotoxic antibody response. *J. nat. Cancer Inst.*, **46**, 391-396 (1971).

IRLIN, I. S., Immunofluorescent demonstration of a specific surface antigen in cells infected or transformed by polyoma virus. *Virology*, **32**, 725-728 (1967).

KIT, S., KURIMURA, T., and DUBBS, D. R., Transplantable mouse tumor line induced by injection of SV40-transformed mouse kidney cells. *Int. J. Cancer*, **4**, 384-392 (1969).

LEVIN, M. J., OXMAN, M. N., DIAMANDOPOULOS, G. Th., LEVINE, A. S., HENRY, P. H., and

ENDERS, J. F., Virus-specific nuclear acids in SV40 exposed hamster embryo cell lines: correlation with S and T antigen. *Proc. nat. Acad. Sci. (Wash.)*, **62**, 589-596 (1969).

LEVINE, A. S., OXMAN, M. N., HENRY, P. H., LEVIN, M. J., DIAMANDOPOULOS, G. Th., and ENDERS, J. F., Virus specific deoxyribonucleic acid in Simian virus 40-exposed hamster cells: correlation with S and T antigens. *J. Virol.*, **6**, 199-207 (1970).

MALMGREN, R. A., TAKEMOTO, K. K., and CARNEY, P. G., Immunofluorescent studies of mouse and hamster cell surface antigens induced by polyoma virus. *J. nat. Cancer Inst.*, **40**, 263-268 (1968).

SMITH, R. W., MORGANROTH, J., and MORA, P. T., SV40 virus-induced tumor-specific transplantation antigen in cultured mouse cells. *Nature (Lond.)*, **227**, 141-145 (1970).

SPARKS, F. C., CANTY, T. G., TING, C. C., HAMMOND, W. G., and HERBERMAN, R. B., Antibody response to skin allografts in mice. *Proc. Soc. exp. Biol. (N.Y.)*, **133**, 1392-1396 (1970).

SPARKS, F. C., TING, C. C., HAMMOND, W. G., and HERBERMAN, R. B., An isotopic antiglobulin technique for measuring antibodies to cell-surface antigen. *J. Immunol.*, **102**, 842-847 (1969).

TAKEMOTO, K. K., MALMGREN, R. A., and HABEL, K., Heat-labile serum factor required for immunofluorescence of polyoma tumor antigen. *Science*, **153**, 1122-1123 (1966).

TAKEMOTO, K. K., TING, R. C. Y., OZER, H. L., and FABISCH, P., Establishment of a cell line from an inbred mouse strain for viral transformation studies: Simian virus 40 transformation and tumor production. *J. nat. Cancer Inst.*, **41**, 1401-1409 (1968).

TEVETHIA, S. S., DIAMANDOPOULOS, G. Th., RAPP, F., and ENDERS, J. F., Lack of relationship between virus-specific surface and transplantation antigens in hamster cells transformed by Simian virus SV40. *J. Immunol.*, **101**, 1192-1198 (1968).

TEVETHIA, S. S., KATZ, M., and RAPP, F., New surface antigen in cells transformed by Simian papovavirus SV40. *Proc. Soc. exp. Biol. (N.Y.)*, **119**, 896-901 (1965).

TING, C. C., and HERBERMAN, R. B., Detection of humoral antibody response to polyoma tumor specific cell surface antigen. *J. nat. Cancer Inst.*, **44**, 729-737 (1970).

TING, C. C., and HERBERMAN, R. B., Kinetics of the response of different classes of antibodies to skin allografts in mice. *Transplantation*, **11**, 390-395 (1971).

106

Reaction of Serum from Pregnant Hamsters with Surface of Cells Transformed by SV40 [1]

RONALD DUFF AND FRED RAPP

Human adenocarcinomas of the digestive tract contain common "tumor-specific" antigens (1). These antigens have also been found to cross-react with antigens found in embryonic and fetal tissue but not with normal tissue (2). Sera from pregnant women appear to contain antibodies directed against these antigens (Gold, personal communication). Hamster cells which have been transformed by simian virus 40 (SV40) have a surface (S) antigen which has been found to be specific for cells transformed by the virus (3). This report describes observations that suggest that the surface antigen on SV40-transformed Syrian hamster cells may be immunologically related to an antigen found during embryonic development.

MATERIALS AND METHODS

Immunofluorescence techniques for the detection of SV40 S antigen have been previously described (3, 4). Antisera reacting specifically with the S antigen were prepared by two methods. In the first method weanling hamsters (Con Olsen) were injected with 10^6 SV40-transformed marmoset monkey cells at weekly intervals for 4 weeks. Five weeks after the initial injection, the animals were bled by cardiac puncture and the sera were collected and pooled. The second method utilized SV40 virus which had been purified by density gradient centrifugation in cesium chloride. Weanling hamsters were injected five times at weekly intervals with 10^{10} viral particles and bled by cardiac puncture 7 weeks after the initial injection.

RESULTS

Sera from pregnant hamsters 14 or 15 days after onset of their second pregnancy were collected and reacted with cells transformed by SV40 or by

[1] This work was supported by Contract NIH 70-2024 from the National Institutes of Health, Department of Health, Education and Welfare.

PARA (defective SV40)-adenovirus 7 (Ad 7), or with spontaneously transformed hamster cells. As shown in Table I, the majority (greater than 80%) of the pregnant hamster sera reacted specifically with the surface of cells transformed by the SV40 genome. No reaction was observed with normal cells or with the spontaneously transformed cells.

The specificity of the pregnant sera for cells transformed by SV40 is also demonstrated in Table II. In this experiment, pregnant sera which reacted with SV40- and PARA-transformed cells did not react with hamster cells transformed by simian adenovirus 7 or by dimethylbenzanthracene (DMBA), or with either spontaneously transformed cells or normal hamster embryo fibroblasts. Furthermore, antisera specifically prepared against the SV40 S antigen reacted in an identical manner and served as the positive control. Serum from female hamsters known never to have been pregnant did not react with the surface of any of the cell types tested.

The correlation of the appearance of this S antibody with the gravid state of the animal is shown in Table III. Sera from weanling female hamsters which did not react with the surface of the SV40-transformed cells were a negative control. Sera from hamsters which were 3 to 5 days pregnant for the first time did not contain anti-S antibodies. The surface reaction occurred in only one of seven sera from initially gravid hamsters, 13 to 15 days after impregnation. The results with second pregnancy hamsters were in contrast to those obtained with first pregnancy hamsters. One of three sera collected 3 to 5 days after impregnation contained antibodies against the S antigen. However, five of six sera were positive when the hamsters were 13 to 15 days pregnant for the second time.

The persistence of the antibody in hamsters after the termination of pregnancy was found to be limited. It was not detectable 1 week after

TABLE I

Surface reaction with sera from gravid hamsters against transformed hamster cells carrying the SV40 genome

Cell Type	Positive Sera	Negative Sera	Per Cent Positive	Per Cent Negative
SV40-transformed (H-50)[a]	22	4	85	15
PARA-Ad7 transformed (1e)[b]	25	5	83	17
PARA-Ad7 transformed (2cT-1)[c]	23	5	82	18
Hamster embryo[d] fibroblasts	0	31	0	100
BHK-21[e]	0	14	0	100

[a] The H-50 cells were from a tumor induced by the injection of SV40 into a newborn Syrian hamster. They have been carried for 28 to 35 passages in cell culture.

[b] The 1e cells were transformed by PARA-Ad7 in vitro. These cells have been shown to be oncogenic in weanling hamsters. The 1e cells were in tissue culture passage 35 to 45.

[c] The 2cT-1 cells were transformed by a variant of PARA-Ad7 which induces the SV40-tumor antigen in the cytoplasm. The 2cT-1 cells were in tissue culture passage 36 to 38.

[d] The hamster embryo fibroblasts were from 14-day hamster embryos and were used in tissue culture passage 1.

[e] A spontaneously transformed line of baby hamster kidney cells.

delivery and did not reappear during the ensuing 5 weeks in which the animals were tested. Dilution of the positive sera yielded negative results; therefore, slight loss in titer following termination of pregnancy may account for this rapid loss of activity.

DISCUSSION

The results presented in the paper show that sera from pregnant hamsters may contain antibodies which react with an antigen on the surface of hamster cells transformed by SV40. Preliminary results indicate that the reaction is specific for SV40-transformed cells and that normal hamster cells, as well as SA7, DMBA, and spontaneously transformed cells do not have this antigen on their surface. Neither a direct nor an indirect relationship of a fetal antigen to the previously described SV40 S antigen has been demonstrated. However, it has been shown by

other investigators that the presence of the SV40 genome is not necessary for the presence of SV40 S antigen on transformed cells (5). The loss of the viral genome from the cell without loss of a specific antigen may indicate that the antigen

TABLE II

Specificity of the surface reaction of pregnant hamster sera for transformed cells containing the SV40 genome

Type of Serum	Cells Transformed by					
	SV40	PARA	SA7[a]	DMBA	Spont.	None[b]
Pg. hamster	+	+	−	−	−	−
Pg. hamster	+	+	−	−	−	−
Pg. hamster	+	+	−	−	−	−
Anti-SV40 S[c]	+	+	−	−	−	−
Anti-SV40 S[d]	+	+	−	−	−	−
Nor. hamster[e]	−	−	−	−	−	−
Nor. hamster	−	−	−	−	−	−

[a] SA7, simian adenovirus 7.

[b] None, hamster embryo fibroblasts.

[c] Antiserum prepared by injection of transformed marmoset cells, see Materials and Methods.

[d] Antiserum prepared by injection of purified SV40, see Materials and Methods.

[e] Nor. hamster: sera from 3-month-old female hamsters.

TABLE III

Correlation of the surface reaction with the gravid state of the hamster

Pregnant State of the Animal	Days after Impregnation	Cell Type		
		AHK[a]	H-5[b]	PARA-Ad7 (1e)[c]
Weanling female hamster	0	0/7[d]	0/7	0/7
First pregnancy	3–5	0/3	0/3	0/3
First pregnancy	13–15	0/7	1/7	1/7
Second pregnancy	3–5	0/3	1/3	1/3
Second pregnancy	13–15	0/6	5/6	5/6

[a] AHK: adult hamster kidney cells, tissue culture passage number 1.

[b] H-50: cells from a tumor induced by SV40 in a newborn Syrian hamster. Animal passage number 4 and tissue culture passage number 25.

[c] 1e: hamster cells transformed in vitro by the PARA-Ad7 hybrid, tissue culture passage number 30.

[d] Number sera positive/number sera tested.

represents the expression of a cellular gene, which might be normally expressed during embryonic development.

A second alternative is suggested by the possibility that the surface antigen detected with sera from pregnant hamsters is one of a mosaic of antigens found on the surface of a cell following transformation by SV40. Some of these antigens may represent the derepression of cellular genes, and other surface antigens may be the result of gene products from the SV40 genome itself.

REFERENCES

1. Gold, P. and Freedman, S. O., J. Exp. Med., *121:* 439, 1965.
2. Gold, P. and Freedman, S. O., J. Exp. Med., *122:* 467, 1965.
3. Tevethia, S. S., Katz, M. and Rapp, F., Proc. Soc. Exp. Biol. Med., *119:* 896, 1965.
4. Duff, R. and Rapp, F., J. Virol., In press.
5. Levin, M. J., Oxman, M. N., Diamandopoulos, G. T., Levine, A. S., Henry, P. H. and Enders, J. F., Proc. Nat. Acad. Sci., *62:* 589, 1969.

Cell-Surface Changes after Infection with Oncogenic Viruses: Requirement for Synthesis of Host DNA

JOHN R. SHEPPARD
ARNOLD J. LEVINE
MAX M. BURGER

Cultured animal cells that have undergone transformation by virus are characterized by a variety of changes when compared to the noninfected parent cell (1). The changes in cell surface may alter the growth characteristics of infected cells (2). Changes in the antigenic (3) and chemical (4) properties of the transformed cell surface have been reported, and some of them can be correlated with the loss of growth control (5).

The agglutinability of almost all permanently transformed cells is increased by pure wheat germ agglutinin (WGA), in comparison with that of noninfected parent cells (6, 7). The WGA surface receptor site, which is present in normal cells in a cryptic form, may be exposed by brief treatment with proteolytic enzymes (7); it was recently demonstrated that surface receptors for another agglutinin, as well as for tumor antigens, are also components of normal cell surfaces and that they become exposed in transformed cells (8).

Other results indicated that the WGA site was exposed approximately 72 hours after the 3T3 cells were infected with SV40 virus (abortive infection). These results were confirmed by data obtained from similar experiments with a permissive virus infection (9).

While studying the appearance of a surface change during lytic infection and abortive transformation, we found that the surface structure was changed only when a virus-directed or -induced synthesis of host DNA occurred after infection. Division of 3T3 cells (abortive infection) has been reported to be a requirement for the exposure of an agglutinin site after viral infection (10). We now present evidence that virus-directed or -induced synthesis of DNA is required for the cell surface alteration that occurs after viral infection.

Figure 1 shows that in both lytic infection (SV40/CV-1, Ad-5/CV-1, Ad-5/BSC-1) and abortive transformation (SV40/3T3) agglutinability increased five- to tenfold within 24 to 72 hours after infection. The WGA site was exposed in the monkey cell lines BSC-1 and CV-1 24 to 30 hours after infection with adenovirus. These cells, however, showed quite different reactions to SV40 infection: the WGA site in CV-1 cells was exposed as with adenovirus, but at a later time (40 hours); the WGA site was not exposed at all in the BSC-1 cells (11), even after 120 hours, at which time a cytopathic effect was evident.

Although the WGA site in BSC-1 cells was not exposed after SV40 in-

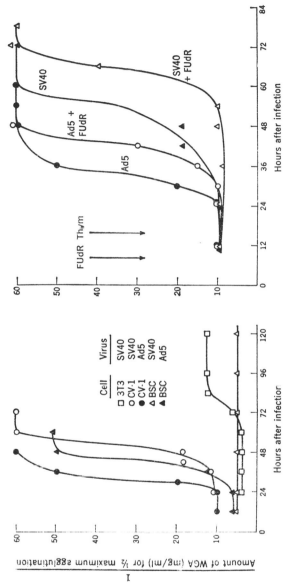

Fig. 1 (left). Time course of agglutinability of cells infected by SV40 or adenovirus. All cell cultures were maintained at 37°C in plastic petri dishes (100 cm²) containing modified Eagle's medium supplemented with calf serum (10 percent) and penicillin-streptomycin (1 percent) as modified by Smith *et al.* (17). Wild-type SV40 and type 5 adenovirus (*Ad*) were used in multiplicities of infection from 50 to 100. After absorption of the virus for 2 hours, the cells were washed twice with medium. In mock infections (controls) the virus was omitted. The agglutination assay has been described (13). Half maximum agglutination is the point where 75 percent of the cells have exposed surface sites (= 2 + on a scale from 0 to 4 +); therefore some cells must have undergone this cell surface change before the first increase visible on the graph occurred. Agglutination after infection was not just the result of release of proteolytic enzymes from the damaged surface, since medium collected from BSC-1 cells 48 hours after infection with adenovirus did not cause exposure of WGA sites on uninfected BSC-1 cells. Fig. 2 (right). Time course of agglutinability of CV-1 cells. DNA synthesis was inhibited by FUdR at a final concentration of $2 \times 10^{-6}M$ added 8 hours after infection. The medium was changed 18 hours after infection, and the cells were rinsed once with medium and then with medium supplemented with $10^{-6}M$ thymidine (*Thym*). Similar results were obtained with 5×10^{-3} and $1 \times 10^{-2}M$ hydroxyurea, which is known to specifically inhibit the formation of deoxyribonucleotides from ribonucleotides (18) and thereby interfere with DNA synthesis before any other macromolecular synthesis.

fection, exposure is possible since the site was exposed after infection with adenovirus. The site can also be exposed by brief treatment of the cell surface with trypsin 60 hours after infection. Agglutination after treatment with trypsin was quantitatively and qualitatively [N-acetylglucosamine inhibition (6)] identical with agglutination in adenovirus infected cells.

Viral infection usually induces or increases the rate of DNA synthesis in the host cell; however, no such synthesis is induced by infection of BSC-1 cells with SV40 (12). Figure 1 shows that the only cell in which the WGA site was not exposed after SV40 infection was also the BSC-1 cell. Since there was potential for exposure of the WGA site after infection of the BSC-1 line with another virus (adenovirus), which also transiently induced host DNA synthesis, we designed experiments to answer the question whether inhibition of DNA synthesis would prevent exposure of the WGA site after infection (Fig. 2).

Infection of CV-1 cells by adenovirus or SV40 would normally lead to exposure of the WGA site after 30 and 40 hours, respectively. An inhibitor of DNA synthesis added 8 hours after infection and maintained for 10 hours delayed exposure of the WGA site (Fig. 2). Similar results have been observed when fluorodeoxyuridine (FUdR) and hydroxyurea were used as inhibitors of DNA synthesis in 3T3 cells infected with polyoma virus (13, 14).

These results, together with those obtained when BSC-1 cells were infected with SV40, indicate that synthesis of host DNA is required for the observed change in the cell surface. The alternative interpretation that synthesis of viral DNA is required can be rejected for the following reasons:

1) Little or no SV40 viral DNA is synthesized in 3T3 cells, but the cell surface site is exposed (Fig. 1).

2) A temperature-sensitive mutant of polyoma virus causes exposure of the site under conditions in which viral DNA is not synthesized (Py-ts 616) (14).

3) That synthesis of host DNA is required for the cell surface change after infection is also supported by experiments with another BSC-1 cell line (15), which was different from the one used in our study. In these other cells in which the synthesis of DNA was induced with SV40, the WGA site was exposed by 36 hours after infection, as predicted. Results of studies with this second cell line, which bears the designation BSC-1 but which appears to be a different line, are in agreement with the results of studies of the inhibition of host-DNA synthesis after viral infection.

Benjamin's host-range mutant of polyoma virus (16) has been shown to initiate DNA synthesis in 3T3 cells without the subsequent exposure of the WGA sites. But exposure of the site has not been demonstrated in the absence of previous DNA synthesis. These results indicate that DNA synthesis is necessary for the appearance of the cell surface alteration but that DNA synthesis alone does not ensure exposure of WGA sites after infection with an oncogenic virus.

We conclude that (i) transformation, lytic infection, and abortive transformation lead to the agglutinable state of the cell surface; and, that (ii) synthesis of host DNA appears to be necessary for the alteration in the surface of the membrane brought about by infection with oncogenic viruses.

1. R. Dulbecco, *Science* 166, 962 (1969).
2. M. M. Burger, in *Growth Control in Cell Cultures* (Little, Brown, Boston, in press).
3. K. Habel, *Proc. Soc. Exp. Biol. Med.* 106, 722 (1961); H. O. Sjögren, J. Hellström, G. Klein, *Cancer Res.* 21. 329 (1961).
4. S. Hakomori and W. G. Murakami, *Proc. Nat. Acad. Sci. U.S.* 59, 254 (1968); N. Ohta, A. B. Pardee, B. R. McAuslan, M. M. Burger, *Biochim. Biophys. Acta* 158, 98 (1968); H. C. Wu, E. Meezan, P. H. Black, P. W. Robbins, *Biochemistry* 8, 2509 (1969).
5. R. E. Pollack and M. M. Burger, *Proc. Nat. Acad. Sci. U.S.* 62, 1074 (1969); M. M. Burger and K. D. Noonan. *Nature* 228, 512 (1970).
6. M. M. Burger and A. R. Goldberg, *Proc. Nat. Acad. Sci. U.S.* 57, 359 (1967).
7. M. M. Burger, *ibid.* 62, 994 (1969).
8. M. Inbar and L. Sachs, *ibid.* 63, 1418 (1969); P. Häyry and V. Defendi, *Virology* 41, 22 (1970).
9. M. M. Burger, M. Inbar, L. Sachs, in preparation.
10. H. Ben-Bassat, M. Inbar, L. Sachs, *Virology* 40, 854 (1970).
11. From D. R. E. Pollack.
12. D. Gershon, L. Sachs, E. Winocour, *Proc. Nat. Acad. Sci. U.S.* 56, 918 (1966); E. Ritzi and A. J. Levine, *J. Virol.* 6, 686 (1970).
13. T. Benjamin and M. M. Burger, *Proc. Nat. Acad. Sci. U.S.* 67, 929 (1970).
14. W. Eckhart, R. Dulbecco, M. M. Burger, *ibid.* 68, 283 (1971).
15. From Dr. T. Benjamin.
16. T. Benjamin, *Proc. Nat. Acad. Sci. U.S.* 67, 394 (1970).
17. J. D. Smith, G. Freeman, M. Vogt, R. Dulbecco, *Virology* 12, 185 (1960).
18. I. H. Krakoff, N. C. Brown, P. Reichard, *Cancer Res.* 28, 1559 (1968).
19. This work was supported by PHS grants CA10151, K4-CA16,765, GM45617, and CA-11049 and by grants P-450 and E-591 from the American Cancer Society.

Cellular Response to SV-40 Infection

Biochemical Consequences of Type 2 Adenovirus and Simian Virus 40 Double Infections of African Green Monkey Kidney Cells

MICHAEL P. FRIEDMAN, MICHAEL J. LYONS, AND HAROLD S. GINSBERG

Rabson et al. reported that simian virus 40 (SV_{40}) facilitated the replication of types 5 and 12 adenovirus in African green monkey kidney (AGMK) cells which are normally restrictive for the multiplication of human adenoviruses (32). Enhancement of adenovirus replication was dependent on prior or simultaneous infection of the cells with SV_{40} (28, 32). Other investigators (34) extended the list of human adenoviruses whose propagation SV_{40} enhanced in AGMK cells, making it appear likely that most, if not all, human adenoviruses could engage in this functional interaction with an unrelated virus. Enhancement was not found when other deoxyribonucleic acid (DNA) viruses were substituted for SV_{40} (11, 28).

Subsequent studies showed that human adenoviruses undergo an abortive replicative cycle in AGMK cells (11). Under conditions of single infection, early adenovirus antigens could be detected by immunofluorescence (11, 25) from

which it became apparent that the initial stages of the replicative cycle, involving adsorption, penetration, and uncoating of the infecting virions, are unaffected. Analyses of DNA extracted from singly and doubly infected cultures revealed that adenovirus DNA is synthesized during abortive infections (33, 35). Similarly, Baum et al. (2) extracted adenovirus-specific ribonucleic acid (mRNA) from singly and doubly infected cells, but the nature of the mRNA detected by hybridization (i.e., early or late) was not investigated.

Under the conditions described, adenoviruses in some respects operationally resemble a conditionally lethal or defective mutant in which the AGMK cell is a nonpermissive host. SV_{40}, a genetically unrelated virus, serves a helper function which permits multiplication of the otherwise "defective" virus. In the absence of well-characterized adenovirus mutants, it seemed possible that adenoviruses in AGMK cells

116

might serve as a substitute that could help reveal some of the factors which regulate the sequential synthesis of adenovirus gene products. The present report describes experiments designed to investigate further the nature of the restriction imposed on propagation of human adenoviruses in AGMK cells and to assess the role SV_{40} plays in converting the abortive infection into a productive one.

MATERIALS AND METHODS

Viruses. The prototype strain of type 2 adenovirus, which was used in the experiments to be described, was plaque-purified three times and shown to be free from adeno-associated virus (AAV) by complement-fixation and electron microscopic techniques. KB cell spinner cultures were infected to prepare pools of adenovirus as previously described (23). The SV_{40} virus (kindly supplied by A. Girardi, Wistar Institute) was also plaque-purified three times in CV-1 cells. SV_{40} was prepared in roller-bottle cultures of CV-1 cells infected with 0.1 plaque-forming unit (PFU)/cell and harvested when the cell sheet revealed 2 + cytopathic effects. The cell suspension was concentrated 10- to 20-fold and sonically treated (Measuring & Scientific Co. Ltd., ultrasonic disintegrator) for 1 min.

Tissue culture. KB cells were propagated in spinner cultures employing minimal essential medium (MEM) supplemented with 10% calf serum. Monolayers of KB cells were also prepared in 35-mm plastic petri dishes with the same medium; for infection of monolayer cultures, MEM supplemented with 5% calf serum was used (10).

Primary AGMK cells were purchased from Flow Laboratories, Rockville, Md., and grown in basal Eagle medium containing 5% fetal calf serum.

Infectivity assay. Adenovirus was assayed on monolayers of KB cells by the plaque assay previously described (23). SV_{40} was assayed in monolayers of AGMK cells by using the same procedure, except that 15% fetal calf serum was present in the overlay. The fluorescent focus assay of Philipson (30) revised by Thiel and Smith (39) was also employed for titration of adenovirus. The Zeiss G.F.L. microscope illuminated by an Osram HBO 200-w mercury lamp was fitted with a 5-mm grid in one ocular to facilitate focus counting. Fluorescein-conjugated goat anti-rabbit gamma globulin (Hyland Laboratories, Los Angeles, Calif.) and rhodamine bovine albumin (Microbiological Associates, Bethesda, Md.) were employed in the indirect technique.

Immunofluorescence of "early" viral antigens. AGMK cells, grown to confluence on cover slips (9 by 22 mm) were infected with the appropriate virus or viruses. To insure that late adenovirus antigens were not produced, 5-fluoro-2-deoxyuridine (FUdR; Hoffman-LaRoche, Nutley, N.J.), at a final concentration of 5×10^{-6} M, was added to the medium after viral adsorption and again 24 hr after infection. The cover slips were rinsed in 0.15 M NaCl buffered with 0.01 M phosphate [pH 7.2 (PBS)] 36 or 48 hr postinfection and fixed in cold acetone at

−20 C for 10 min. The SV_{40} virus-infected cells were stained with fluorescein-tagged pooled gamma globulin from hamsters bearing SV_{40}-induced tumors (Flow Laboratories, Inc.). Specific rabbit antisera against early or late adenovirus antigen(s) (14, 36) were used in the indirect fluorescent-antibody proprocedure. All specimens, including uninfected control slides, were examined under an oil immersion apochromatic objective (40 ×).

Complement fixation. A microtechnique was employed (37). Antigen titers are expressed as the highest dilution that completely fixed 2 units of guinea pig complement in the presence of 4 to 8 units of antibody.

Preparation of antisera. Rabbits were immunized with purified type 5 adenovirus hexon (24), purified type 2 adenovirus, or a homogenate prepared from cells infected with type 2 adenovirus in the presence of 5×10^{-5} M FUdR and harvested 16 hr after infection. This latter inoculum was tested for the presence of infectious virus, and, after immunization, the antisera obtained were examined for the presence of antibody against late viral proteins. In each instance, the immunizing material was mixed with Freund's adjuvant and injected in 0.5-ml quantities into the four foot pads. One month later, each rabbit received 0.1 ml safe of admunin in the adjuvant suspension and was bled 10 days afterwards.

Autoradiography. Confluent cultures of AGMK cells on cover slips were infected with virus; others were mock-infected and served as controls. Eighteen hours after infection, 0.2 μc of ³H-thymidine per ml (thymidine-*methyl-³H*, 3.6 mc/mg, New England Nuclear Corp., Boston, Mass.) was added to the maintenance medium. The medium was removed 30 hr after infection, and the cell sheets were washed three times with PBS and fixed in ethanol-glacial acetic acid (3:1, v/v) for 10 min at room temperature. The cultures were washed successively in 70, 40, 20, and 10% aqueous ethanol washes, rinsed in distilled water, and extracted twice with cold 5% trichloroacetic acid for 10 min (1). The cultures were then rinsed in distilled water, 70% ethanol, and 95% ethanol and allowed to air-dry before being mounted on microscope slides. The fixed cultures were dipped in 44% NTB2 emulsion (Kodak), dried for 1 hr, and stored at 4 C for 7 days. After development, the slides were stained with hematoxylin and eosin and each was studied microscopically to determine the proportion of cells containing isotope and the number of grains per nucleus. A minimum of 1,000 cells were counted per preparation. Uninfected cells to which ³H-thymidine had not been added were examined as emulsion control preparations; less than three grains per cell were found.

Preparation of ³H-labeled SV_{40} DNA. To each confluent culture of CV-1 cells in production roller bottles, SV_{40} at a multiplicity of approximately 0.1 PFU/cell was added in 10 ml of infecting fluid. After 2 hr at 37 C, 200 ml of maintenance medium was added to each culture. ³H-thymidine (0.5 μc per ml of medium) was added 24 hr postinfection. At 6 to 7 days after infection, when greater than 50% of the cells showed cytopathic effects, the cells were scraped

117

into the medium and sedimented by centrifugation. Virus was purified by the procedure of Black et al. (5) by employing two equilibrium density gradient centrifugations in CsCl. After dialysis against tris(hydroxymethyl)aminomethane (Tris)-buffered saline (Tris-hydrochloride, 0.01 M, pH 8.1; NaCl, 0.15 M), the viral DNA was extracted by the method of Watson and Littlefield (42). The DNA obtained had a specific activity of 6,250 counts per min per μg of DNA, consisted of a single 20S peak after band centrifugation in CsCl (41), and was eluted in a single peak from a methylated albumin-kieselguhr (MAK) column (26) at 0.55 M NaCl.

Purification of adenovirus and extraction of viral DNA. After preliminary preparation, virus was purified by centrifugation in CsCl gradients and the DNA was obtained as previously described (4, 24).

Preparation of labeled DNA from virus-infected and uninfected cells. AGMK cells were grown to confluence in roller bottles; some cultures were not infected, and the remaining ones were infected with adenovirus or adenovirus and SV$_{40}$ virus. Sixteen hours after infection, ^{3}H-thymidine (1 μc per ml of medium) was added to each bottle; the cultures were incubated for 20 hr after which the cells were harvested and washed. DNA was extracted by a procedure similar to that employed by Reich et al. (35). Approximately 10^8 cells were suspended in 2 ml of a buffer containing 0.1 M NaCl, 0.01 M ethylenediaminetetraacetic acid (EDTA), 0.05 M Tris-hydrochloride (pH 8.6), and 0.5% sodium dodecyl sulfate (SDS). Freshly prepared Pronase (Calbiochem, grade B, 45,000 PUK/g) was added to give a final concentration of 1 mg/ml, and the suspensions were incubated at 37 C with intermittent gentle shaking for 2 to 3 hr or overnight at room temperature. After two to three extractions with 80% freshly distilled phenol, the DNA solution was extracted once with anhydrous ether and dialyzed against 0.1 SSC (0.15 M NaCl plus 0.015 M sodium citrate) at 4 C for 24 to 48 hr, with at least three changes of buffer. A few drops of chloroform were added to the DNA and it was stored at 4 C. This procedure recovered approximately 90% of the DNA.

Selective extraction of viral DNA. Confluent monolayer cultures of AGMK cells in 60-mm plastic petri dishes were infected with adenovirus, SV$_{40}$ virus, or combinations of both viruses. In each experiment, cultures were also mock-infected. Three cultures were employed for each group. After infection, spent medium (from 1- to 2-day-old cultures) was added. After 16 hr of incubation at 37 C in a CO$_2$ incubator, 10 μc of ^{3}H-thymidine or ^{14}C-thymidine was added to each plate. Thirty-six hours after infection, the medium was discarded and the cell sheets were washed once with PBS. A 1-ml amount of 0.6% SDS in 0.01 M EDTA, 0.01 M Tris-hydrochloride (pH 8.1) was added to each plate, and the viral DNA was extracted by the method of Hirt (20) for the separation of polyoma virus DNA from host nuclear DNA. To determine the proportion of adenovirus or SV$_{40}$ virus DNA not extracted in the selective procedure, the pellets were treated with Pronase and the DNA was extracted three times with chloroform-isoamyl alcohol (24:1) as in the procedure of Marmur (27)

or with 80% phenol. The types of DNA were analyzed by isopycnic gradient centrifugation in CsCl. The selective extraction procedure was found to recover 95% of the adenovirus and SV$_{40}$ DNA from infected cells.

To determine the quantity of host DNA extracted in the selective procedure described above, growing cells were labeled with ^{3}H-thymidine until confluent monolayers were obtained. Cold medium was substituted for the radioactive medium for 24 hr to deplete the ^{3}H-thymidine cellular pool. The cultures were subsequently infected and labeled with ^{14}C-thymidine; 36 hr after infection, the DNA was extracted as described above. A portion of each extract was subjected to rate zonal centrifugation, and the ^{3}H and ^{14}C content of each fraction was determined. No significant level of ^{3}H counts was observed.

Sedimentation analysis (band centrifugation) of DNA. A 10- to 20-μg amount of DNA in 0.2 ml was layered onto 3 ml of CsCl (Harshaw Chemical Co., optical grade) having a density of 1.5 g/ml in 0.01 M EDTA, 0.01 M Tris-hydrochloride (pH 8.1) and was centrifuged in a Spinco SW 39 rotor at 99,972 $\times$ g for 3.25 hr at 20 C (9, 41). Fractions (two drops) were collected from the bottom of the tubes onto Whatman no. 3 filter-paper discs (2.3 cm). The discs were briefly oven-dried, washed twice with 5% ice-cold trichloroacetic acid for 20 min, washed with acetone, and dried. Radioactivity was assayed in a Packard Tri-Carb liquid scintillation spectrometer using 5 ml of phosphor (40).

Chromatography on MAK columns. MAK was prepared as described by Mandell and Hershey (26). The column (1.9 by 6 cm) was made in a single layer (38), and the adsorbed DNA was eluted in steps with increasing concentrations of NaCl (0.5 to 0.7 M) containing 0.05 M phosphate buffer (pH 6.7). Fractions of 5 ml were collected and 0.1 ml of each was spotted on a filter-paper disc for assay in a scintillation spectrometer (40). DNA was also measured by optical density at 260 nm and by the diphenylamine reaction (6).

Isopycnic gradient centrifugation. DNA samples were layered on 4 ml of CsCl solution having a density of 1.7 g/ml in Tris-hydrochloride-EDTA buffer (pH 8.1) and were centrifuged in the Spinco SW 39 rotor for 70 hr at 99,972 $\times$ g at 20 C. Fractions were collected and counted as described above. Fractions at both sides of the peaks were collected under oil for estimation of buoyant density by using an Abbe refractometer.

RESULTS

Multiplication of type 2 adenovirus in AGMK cells in the absence or presence of SV$_{40}$ virus. Adenoviruses reportedly do not multiply in primary monkey kidney cells except in the presence of SV$_{40}$ virus (11, 28, 32). The experiments that described this enhancement phenomenon were carried out with multiplicities of adenovirus which presumably infected less than one-half of the cells (11, 28, 32). However, to investigate biochemically the mechanism by

118

which SV_{40} converts an abortive adenovirus infection into a productive infection, it was desirable to infect all of the cells. Preliminary experiments in which various multiplicities of each virus were employed demonstrated that 30 PFU of SV_{40} per cell produced optimum enhancement of adenovirus multiplication, that maximum enhancement of adenovirus propagation could be detected when a relatively low multiplicity of type 2 adenovirus was employed, and that some adenovirus multiplication ensued, albeit a relatively small amount, when cells were infected with adenovirus alone. The larger the adenovirus inoculum, the greater the amount of adenovirus produced.

An analysis of the multiplication of type 2 adenovirus in AGMK cells in the presence and absence of SV_{40} is summarized in Fig. 1. The yield of adenovirus was enhanced approximately 1,000-fold when multiplicities of 3 PFU of adenovirus per cell and 30 PFU of SV_{40} per cell were added to the cultures. When 30 PFU of adenovirus per cell was used, the viral yield was increased only about 250 times. Although adenovirus propagation was greatly limited under conditions of single infection, some viral production occurred. Moreover, the eclipse period of adenovirus multiplication was similar, approximately 16 hr, whether cells were infected with type 2 adenovirus alone or whether SV_{40} was added to the inoculum.

In addition to assays for infectious virus in the experiments described above, complement-fixation titrations were carried out to compare the

TABLE 1. *Production of adenovirus hexon antigen in AGMK cells infected with type 2 adenovirus alone or infected with SV40 and type 2 adenovirus*

Infected with[a]		Complement-fixation titer[b]			
Adenovirus	SV40	4[c]	24	36	48
PFU/cell	*PFU/cell*				
3		0[d]	4	8	16
3	30	0	16	128	256
30		0	16	16	32
30	30	0	64	128	256
	30	0	0	0	0
		0	0	0	0

[a] Duplicate cultures of AGMK cells were infected. Cells were harvested, washed with PBS, and sonically treated for 1 min.

[b] Reciprocal of the complement-fixation titer. Antibody to purified hexon was employed for the titration.

[c] Hours after infection.

[d] Titer of $<1:2$.

relative amounts of adenovirus capsid proteins made in the restrictive and productive infections. These titrations were done with a serum from rabbits immunized with purified hexon (24) to permit detection of relatively small amounts of viral antigens, because complement fixation did not occur with uninfected cell antigens when this serum was employed. The results of a representative experiment (Table 1) demonstrate that adenovirus hexon protein (17) was made in limited quantities when cells were infected only with type 2 adenovirus, and that SV_{40} infection markedly increased the synthesis of adenovirus capsid protein.

Immunofluorescence assay of cells synthesizing adenovirus early proteins and capsid antigens. Cultures infected with type 2 adenovirus produce relatively small numbers of infectious particles; the amount of virus produced is greatly increased (Fig. 1) when cultures are also infected previously or simultaneously with SV_{40} (25, 28, 32). To understand this phenomenon, it was necessary to determine how many cells were infected when adenovirus alone was added and whether, under conditions of enhanced double infections, more cells synthesized early as well as late (i.e., capsid antigen) proteins. To answer the first query, cells were infected in the presence of 5×10^{-6} M FUdR, and 16 hr later they were examined by using serum from rabbits immunized with KB cells infected with type 2 adenovirus in the presence of FUdR. With a small inoculum of adenovirus alone (i.e., input multiplicity of 3 PFU/cell), early protein could be detected in

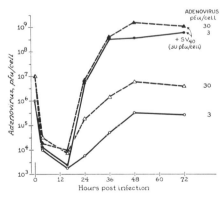

FIG. 1. *Multiplication of type 2 adenovirus in AGMK cells. Monolayers of AGMK cells were infected with adenovirus or adenovirus plus SV_{40}. Replicate cultures were harvested at the times indicated. The washed cell pellets were sonically treated and assayed for adenovirus.*

119

Table 2. *Detection of early adenovirus antigens[a]*
by immunofluorescence

Infected with		Per cent cells positive[b]
Adenovirus	SV40	
PFU/cell	PFU/cell	
3		30
3	30	85–90
30		85–90
30	30	95
	30	0
		0

[a] AGMK cells infected in the presence of 5×10^{-6} M FUdR.

[b] Slides were stained by the indirect method by using rabbit serum containing antibodies to early adenovirus antigens and anti-rabbit goat gamma globulin conjugated with fluorescein isothiocyanate.

Table 3. *Synthesis of early adenovirus antigens*

Infected with		Complement-fixation titer[b]			
Adenovirus[a]	SV40[a]	4[c]	24	36	48
PFU/cell	PFU/cell				
3		0[d]	0	4	4
3	30	0	0	16	16
30		0	0	8	8
30	30	0	8	32	32
	30	0	0	2	2
		0	0	2	2

[a] Infected in the presence of 5×10^{-6} M FUdR.

[b] Complement-fixation test performed using rabbit serum containing antibodies only to early adenovirus antigens. Titer is expressed as the reciprocal. Purified hexon from type 2 adenovirus infected cells did not react with the serum employed.

[c] Hours after infection.

[d] Titer of <1:2.

approximately one-third of the cells (Table 2), but the addition of SV_{40} to the inoculum increased the number of cells showing antigen as well as the intensity of the antigen. Hence, adenovirus could infect almost all of the cells. Although early proteins were detected in only about 30% of the cells when adenovirus alone was used, it is likely that almost all of the cells produced some early proteins and that the addition of SV_{40} either quantitatively or qualitatively altered the synthesis of early proteins so that the immunofluorescence technique easily detected them. Assay of early proteins by complement-fixation assays substantiated the impression that more adenovirus-specific early proteins were made in cells infected with both adenovirus and SV_{40} than when only adenovirus was used as the infecting inoculum (Table 3). It could not be determined whether unique early proteins were made only in the cells infected with both viruses.

Cells were similarly infected in the absence of FUdR to determine in the abortive infection whether each cell was making a small amount of capsid protein or whether only a rare cell was productively infected. It was surprising that 20 to 30% of the cells produced capsid antigens, depending upon the multiplicity of adenovirus infection (Table 4), that the number of cells was only doubled under conditions in which the yield of infectious virus was enhanced 1,000-fold (Fig. 1), and that in cells infected with both viruses the quantity of hexon antigen was only increased about 16-fold (Table 1). Thus, although all cells could be infected with adenovirus, SV_{40} could convert a partially abortive infection into a productive infection in about 50% of the cells; the remainder of the cells were still apparently nonpermissive for propagation of infectious adenovirus.

DNA synthesis in cells infected with type 2 adenovirus or adenovirus and SV_{40}. Since adenovirus can infect all AGMK cells in a culture and adenovirus-specific early proteins can be made

Table 4. *Detection of adenovirus capsid antigens by immunofluorescence[a]*

Infected with		Per cent cells positive[b]
Adenovirus	SV40	
PFU/cell	PFU/cell	
3		22
		20
		20
		23
3	30	39
		39
		41
		42
30		24.5
		31.5
30	30	50
		49
		45
		57

[a] Indirect method with serum from rabbits immunized with purified type 2 adenovirus.

[b] Examined 36 hr after infection.

in the infected cells, it was necessary to determine whether the restriction in synthesis of capsid proteins resulted from a failure to replicate viral DNA in the nonpermissive cells (12) or whether some other biosynthetic step was blocked. To accomplish this objective, DNA synthesis in AGMK cells infected with various multiplicities of adenovirus in the absence or presence of SV_{40} was studied in several ways: (i) incorporation of ^{3}H-thymidine to measure the rate of synthesis of total DNA, (ii) autoradiography to enumerate the number of cells synthesizing DNA, (iii) separation of adenovirus and SV_{40} DNA by velocity centrifugation in CsCl gradients, and (iv) separation of viral from host DNA by chromatography on MAK columns.

Rate of DNA synthesis. At intervals, ^{3}H-thymidine (2 μc/ml) was added for 1 hr to uninfected cells and to cells infected with type 2 adenovirus (3 PFU/cell), with adenovirus (3 PFU/cell) and SV_{40} (30 PFU/cell), or with SV_{40} (30 PFU/cell). The data obtained (Fig. 2) demonstrate that DNA synthesis was markedly increased under each of the conditions of infection, that the rates of DNA synthesis were similar in cells abortively infected with adenovirus or

productively infected when the helper SV_{40} was added, and that infection with SV_{40} alone stimulated DNA synthesis approximately three times more (13, 19, 22) than did adenovirus and SV_{40} together. It should also be noticed that, whereas DNA synthesis attained a maximum rate at 15 to 18 hr after infection with adenovirus or adenovirus and SV_{40}, maximum synthesis occurred approximately 30 hr after SV_{40} infection. This experiment implied that some event in the multiplication of type 2 adenovirus blocked replication of SV_{40} DNA or host DNA, which is enhanced in cells infected only with SV_{40} (13, 19, 22), or that it inhibited the synthesis of both species of DNA. The following analyses were done to clarify this phenomenon.

Separation of adenovirus and SV_{40} DNA by velocity (band) sedimentation in CsCl. Centrifugation (41) of an artificial mixture of type 2 adenovirus DNA and SV_{40} virus DNA extracted from purified viruses sharply separated the two species of viral DNA (Fig. 3). DNA species selectively extracted (20) from cells infected with either virus alone or with both viruses had sedimentation characteristics similar to those of DNA species from purified viruses; conveniently host DNA was not present in the extracted samples. The results of a representative experiment (Fig. 4) demonstrate that (i) synthesis of SV_{40} DNA was increasingly inhibited as the multiplicity of adenovirus infection was increased, (ii) replication of similar quantities of adenovirus DNA occurred in restricted and enhanced infections, and (iii) replication of adenovirus DNA was increased with increasing multiplicities of infecting adenovirus.

Separation of host and viral DNA on MAK

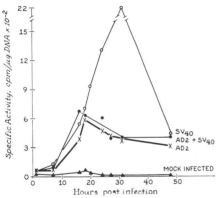

FIG. 2. *Rate of DNA synthesis in AGMK cells infected with type 2 adenovirus or with type 2 adenovirus plus SV_{40}. Confluent monolayers of AGMK cells were infected with type 2 adenovirus (3 PFU/cell), type 2 adenovirus (3 PFU/cell) plus SV_{40} (30 PFU/cell), or SV_{40} alone (30 PFU/cell). Uninfected cultures were studied. At various times after infection, some of the cultures were pulse-labeled with ^{3}H-thymidine (2 μc/ml) for 1 hr and then harvested and washed. The cell pellets were treated with 5% trichloroacetic acid at 4 C. The precipitate was assayed for total DNA and incorporation of ^{3}H-thymidine.*

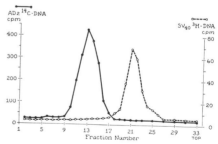

FIG. 3. *Sedimentation analysis of an artificial mixture of type 2 adenovirus ^{14}C-DNA and SV_{40} ^{3}H-DNA. The two species of DNA (10 μg of each in 0.2 ml) were layered onto 3 ml of CsCl (p = 1.5 g/ml) and centrifuged at 99,972 × g for 3.25 hr at 20 C in an SW 39 rotor. Two-drop fractions were collected from the bottom of the tube.*

121

columns. Undenatured SV_{40} and type 2 adenovirus DNA could not be distinguished by chromatography on MAK columns under the conditions employed. Nevertheless, this procedure distinctly separated viral from host-cell DNA, as shown by chromatography of an artificial mixture of type 2 adenovirus and monkey kidney cell DNA (Fig. 5); greater than 90% of the DNA was recovered. It was therefore possible to determine whether adenovirus infection alone or infection in partnership with SV_{40} blocked synthesis of host-cell DNA, and whether the quantity of DNA made in the restricted infection was proportionate to the amount of infectious virus propagated in the enhanced adenovirus-SV_{40} infection. The data obtained from an experiment in which cells were infected only with type 2 adenovirus (Fig. 6) bear upon two of these points: (i) replication of host-cell DNA was blocked and (ii) the quantity of adenovirus DNA synthesized was greatly in excess of either the quantity of virus made in the single infection or the 1,000-fold more virus produced in an enhanced infection. A total of 1.2×10^6 PFU was synthesized in the infected AGMK cells, whereas 72 μg of viral DNA was recovered in the 0.55 M NaCl fractions. If DNA is 13% of the weight of the virion and the virion weighs 2×10^{-16} g (18), then 3.12×10^{-3} μg of DNA was contained in the infectious particles propagated. Even if the assembly of adenovirus in AGMK cells is similar to that in HeLa cells [i.e., only about 10% of the DNA synthesized is incorporated into virions (16)], a very large excess of viral DNA was replicated in the restricted infection as compared to the number of virions assembled.

A similar chromatographic separation was also made on the total DNA extracted from AGMK cells infected with both type 2 adenovirus (10 PFU/cells) and SV_{40} (30 PFU/cell). The data from one such experiment (Fig. 7) demonstrate that biosynthesis of host-cell DNA is not stimulated as it is in cells infected only with SV_{40} (19, 22). A small amount of DNA was eluted in the first fraction of 0.625 M NaCl, but its distribution was not characteristic of normal host-cell DNA. This DNA was not further identified. When DNA eluted from MAK at 0.55 M NaCl was separated by velocity sedimentation in CsCl, it was shown to consist predominantly of adenovirus DNA. Hence, adenovirus infection not only blocked replication of its helper DNA, SV_{40}, but also suppressed the stimulated synthesis of AGMK cell DNA.

Number of cells synthesizing DNA when singly or doubly infected. Autoradiographic techniques were used to determine the number of cells which synthesized DNA under the conditions of infection employed. The data summarized in Fig. 8 reveal that SV_{40} (30 PFU/cell) induced almost all cells to synthesize DNA but that replication of DNA occurred in only about 30% of the cells infected with type 2 adenovirus at a low multiplicity of infection (i.e., 3 PFU/cell), approximately the same number in which production of specific early proteins could be detected. It is striking that infection with 3 PFU of adenovirus per cell and 30 PFU of SV_{40} per cell only increased slightly the number of cells synthesizing DNA as compared to adenovirus alone, although infection with only SV_{40} initiated DNA biosynthesis in practically all of the cells. An inoculum of type 2 adenovirus of 30 or 150 PFU/cell, with or without SV_{40}, caused replication of DNA in almost all of the cells. The experiments also confirmed the evidence presented above (Fig. 2 and 4) that more DNA was made in cells infected only with SV_{40} than in cells doubly infected with SV_{40} and adenovirus except at a very high adenovirus multiplicity (i.e., 150 PFU/cell).

Multiplication of SV_{40} in cells infected with

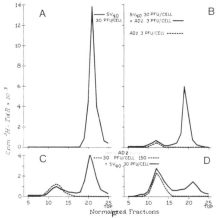

FIG. 4. *Biosynthesis of type 2 adenovirus and SV_{40} DNA in AGMK cells infected with one or both viruses. Three replicate monolayer cultures of AGMK cells were infected with each inoculum: SV_{40}, 30 PFU/cell (A, B, C, D); type 2 adenovirus, 3 PFU/cell (B), 30 PFU/cell (C), or 150 PFU/cell (D). "Spent" medium obtained from the uninfected cultures was added to the cultures after infection. Sixteen hours after infection, 10 μc of ^{3}H-thymidine or ^{14}C-thymidine was added to each culture; 36 hr postinfection the cell sheets were washed three times and viral DNA was selectively extracted. Sedimentation analyses were performed as described in Fig. 3.*

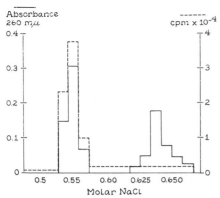

FIG. 5. *Chromatographic separation of an artificial mixture of* [14]*C-labeled type 2 adenovirus DNA and unlabeled, normal monkey kidney cell DNA on a MAK column. Type 2 adenovirus DNA was obtained from purified virus. Approximately 50 μg of each DNA was layered onto the column (1.9 by 6 cm) in 0.2 м NaCl containing 0.05 м phosphate buffer, pH 6.7. Elution was carried out with 0.05 м stepwise increases in NaCl concentration; 5-ml fractions were collected. DNA recovery from the column was greater than 90%.*

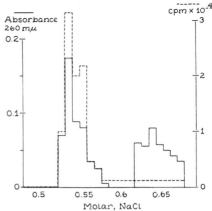

FIG. 6. *Chromatographic separation on MAK column of DNA extracted from AGMK cells infected with type 2 adenovirus. Confluent AGMK cells were infected with type 2 adenovirus, 30 PFU/cell. ^{3}H-thymidine (1 μc/ml) was added 16 hr after infection; the cells were incubated an additional 20 hr and harvested. Cells were disrupted with 0.5% SDS in 0.1 м NaCl, 0.01 м EDTA, and 0.05 м Tris-hydrochloride buffer at pH 8.6, and DNA was extracted as described in Material and Methods. The resultant DNA extract was dialyzed against three changes of 0.2 м NaCl, 0.05 м phosphate buffer (pH 6.7) at 4 C for 48 hr. A 50-μg amount of DNA was added to the MAK column and elution was accomplished as described in Fig. 5. Recovery of DNA was greater than 90%.*

type 2 adenovirus. Biosyntheses of SV_{40} (7) and cellular DNA were markedly decreased in cells concomitantly infected with type 2 adenovirus. It was therefore predicted that production of SV_{40} virions would also be suppressed in cells infected with adenovirus. The results of experiments to test this prediction (Table 5) demonstrate that propagation of SV_{40} was indeed inhibited under conditions in which the multiplication of adenovirus was enhanced. These studies also showed that purified type 2 adenovirus similarly reduced the multiplication of SV_{40} and that crude virus inoculum did not contain sufficient soluble adenovirus antigens (24) to inhibit SV_{40} propagation. In similar experiments, it was also found that greater than 95% of the cells synthesized early SV_{40} T antigen (31), whether infected only with SV_{40} or with both viruses.

Effect of inhibitors of macromolecular synthesis on capacity of SV_{40} to enhance multiplication of type 2 adenovirus. Since type 2 adenovirus inhibited synthesis of SV_{40} DNA and late proteins, although multiplication of adenovirus was enhanced, it seemed probable that an early event in the biosynthesis of SV_{40} was responsible for the increased adenovirus propagation. This possibility was tested by utilizing the finding that the rate of adenovirus multiplication was

distinctly greater in cells infected with SV_{40} 12 to 16 hr before infection with adenovirus than when SV_{40} and adenovirus were added simultaneously (Fig. 9 and 10). Early viral proteins are synthesized in the absence of SV_{40} DNA synthesis (11); it was therefore possible to distinguish whether biosynthesis of SV_{40}-induced early proteins or SV_{40} DNA was necessary to increase adenovirus multiplication in AGMK cells. At the time of infection with SV_{40} (30 PFU/cell), 5×10^{-6} M FUdR was added to stop DNA synthesis. Sixteen hours later, cultures were infected with type 2 adenovirus and excess thymidine (5×10^{-5} M) was added to permit DNA synthesis. The results of a representative experiment (Fig. 9) demonstrate that (i) cells infected with SV_{40} 16 hr before or at the same time as adenovirus produced 200 to 1,000 times more infectious virus than cells infected only with adenovirus, (ii) adenovirus multiplied faster in cells pre-infected with SV_{40} than in cells infected with both viruses simultaneously, and (iii) adenovirus multiplied at the increased rate regardless of whether SV_{40} DNA synthesis oc-

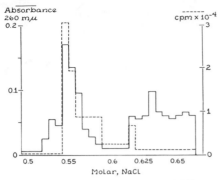

FIG. 7. *Chromatographic separation of DNA extracted from AGMK cells infected with type 2 adenovirus (3 PFU/cell) and SV₄₀ (30 PFU/cell). Procedures for infection, isotopic labeling, extraction of DNA, and MAK chromatography were the same as described in Fig. 5 and 6.*

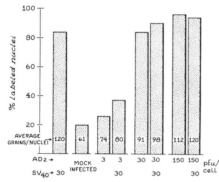

FIG. 8. *Proportion of cells labeled with ³H-thymidine during infection with adenovirus type 2, SV₄₀, or combinations of both viruses. Confluent monolayers of AGMK cells on cover slips were infected; 18 hr after infection, 0.2 μc of ³H-thymidine per ml was added, and the cultures were incubated for an additional 12 hr. Autoradiography was carried out on the cover slips. At least 1,000 cells per preparation were counted.*

curred during the 16 hr before infection with adenovirus.

The data summarized in Fig. 9 strengthen the hypothesis that infection of AGMK cells with SV₄₀ induces the synthesis of a protein which is necessary for propagation of adenovirus, that the protein is not constitutive in the cells, and that its production cannot be brought about by adenovirus. To test this hypothesis directly, cycloheximide (50 μg/ml) was used instead of

TABLE 5. *Effect of infectious adenovirus, inactivated adenovirus, or soluble antigens on multiplication of SV40*

Group	Inoculum		Quantity of SV40[a] produced
	Adenovirus	SV40	
	PFU/cell	PFU/cell	PFU/ml
I	300	30	4.5×10^4
	150	30	1.5×10^5
	30	30	2.5×10^6
	3	30	9.3×10^6
	0	30	2.4×10^7
	Inactivated virus[b]	30	2.4×10^7
	Soluble antigens[c]	30	2.5×10^7
II[d]	150	30	3.5×10^5
	3	30	4.5×10^6
	0	30	2.3×10^7

[a] Infectivity was determined at 48 hr (group I) or 72 hr (group II) after infection.

[b] Hydroxylamine-inactivated adenovirus. Virus was incubated in 1 M hydroxylamine (pH 7.0 to 7.2) at 37 C for 24 hr.

[c] Partially purified mixture of hexon, fiber, and penton. The quantity employed was comparable, as measured in complement-fixation units, to the total amount of soluble antigen inoculated with 300 PFU/cell of crude virus.

[d] Adenovirus in this group was purified.

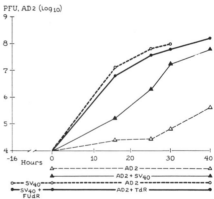

FIG. 9. *Effect of FUdR on the rate of type 2 adenovirus multiplication in cells preinfected with SV₄₀. Two sets of confluent monolayer cultures of AGMK cells (three cultures per set) were infected with SV₄₀ at 30 PFU/cell. After infection, one set received 5 × 10⁻⁶ M FUdR. Sixteen hours after infection, both sets of cultures were infected with adenovirus (30 PFU/cell) and 5 × 10⁻⁶ M thymidine was added to the cultures which received FUdR. Two additional sets of cultures were infected, one with adenovirus and the other with adenovirus and SV₄₀. Replicate cultures of all four sets were assayed for infectious adenovirus.*

124

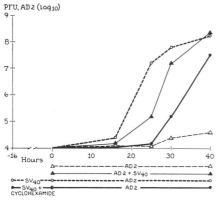

PFU, AD2 (log₁₀)

$$PFU, AD2 \ (log_{10})$$

```
Hours      0    10    20    30    40
Δ----------AD2----------Δ
▲--------- AD2 + SV₄₀ ----------▲
○---SV₄₀---○-----------AD2------------○
●---SV₄₀ +---●---------AD2------------
CYCLOHEXAMIDE
```

Fig. 10. *Effect of cycloheximide on the rate of type 2 adenovirus multiplication in cells preinfected with SV₄₀. Two sets of confluent monolayer cultures of AGMK cells were infected with SV₄₀ (30 PFU/cells); 50 μg of cycloheximide per ml was added to one set of cultures. Sixteen hours after infection, cycloheximide was removed and both groups of cultures were infected with type 2 adenovirus, 30 PFU/cell. Two other groups of cultures were also infected at the same time with type 2 adenovirus and adenovirus plus SV₄₀. Three replicate cultures from each of the four sets were assayed for infectious type 2 adenovirus.*

5-FUdR to inhibit protein synthesis. Sixteen hours after SV₄₀ infection and the addition of cycloheximide, the cultures were washed to remove the inhibitor from the affected cells and adenovirus was added. The results obtained (Fig. 10) demonstrate that, in the absence of protein synthesis, preinfection with SV₄₀ did not increase the rate of adenovirus multiplication. The somewhat retarded appearance of adenovirus in cultures which had received cycloheximide reflects the delay in reversing the effect of the chemical on protein synthesis.

DISCUSSION

AGMK cells are restrictive hosts for adenovirus multiplication (28, 32) although a relatively small number of virions can be formed. The limiting event is not concerned with the initial events in infection of the cell since, except with low viral multiplicities, almost all cells can synthesize virus-specific early proteins. Nevertheless, the quantity of early proteins, and possibly even the number of early proteins, is increased when cells are concomitantly infected with SV₄₀ and adenoviruses. Clearly the synthesis of capsid proteins is the major restriction in abortive adenovirus infection of AGMK cells. Even when co-infected with SV₄₀, approximately one-half the cells do not become permissive for complete adenovirus multiplication, but practically all cells synthesize DNA, the number of virions made is increased approximately 1,000-fold, and the production of capsid proteins is greatly augmented.

Because biosynthesis of adenovirus capsid proteins is dependent upon prior replication of viral DNA (12), it seemed possible that quantitatively viral DNA was limited in the singly infected cells. It had been reported that adenovirus DNA was synthesized even in the abortive infection (33), and Reich et al., with hybridization techniques, showed that in cells infected only with adenovirus approximately one-half the amount of adenovirus DNA was replicated as in cells infected with both viruses (35). Utilizing ultracentrifugation and chromatographic procedures, which permitted identification and quantitative recovery of the three species of DNA concerned, it was possible to demonstrate that approximately the same amount of adenovirus DNA was synthesized in the restricted as in the permissive infection, and that the quantity of viral DNA made was even far in excess of that essential for the number of virions assembled in the enhanced infection.

Investigation of the biosynthesis of DNA in singly and doubly infected cells revealed, however, that the viral interactions were more complicated than anticipated. As compared to a cell infected with SV₄₀ alone, the kinetics of synthesis and the specific activity of the DNA were greatly altered in cells infected simultaneously with SV₄₀ and adenovirus. Quantitative analyses of the species of DNA replicated in the singly and doubly infected cells revealed the basis for these striking alterations in cells infected with both viruses. (i) Synthesis of host DNA was not stimulated as in cells infected only with SV₄₀. (ii) Replication of SV₄₀ DNA was inhibited, the degree of inhibition being dependent upon the multiplicity of adenovirus employed. (iii) Biosynthesis of adenovirus DNA was proportionate to the multiplicity of adenovirus infection and was similar to the amount synthesized in cells infected only with adenovirus.

The molecular basis is unknown for the biochemical conflict which blocks biosynthesis of both host and SV₄₀ DNA while adenovirus DNA is replicated. It seems likely that the synthesis of host DNA is inhibited by a mechanism similar to the switch-off of host DNA synthesis in KB cells productively infected with type 5 adenovirus (15). Although the physical structure of SV₄₀ DNA is strikingly different from that of mammalian cell DNA, the average base composition does not vary greatly; it is possible that the replication of both species of DNA is inhibited by the same mechanism which is specified by the overall base structure or by certain similar nucleotide sequences. Alternatively, it is possible that initiation of SV_{40} DNA is a prerequisite for the enhanced synthesis of host-cell DNA. Hence, if the biosynthesis of SV_{40} DNA is inhibited, the increased synthesis of host DNA is not induced. However, in cells infected with adenovirus alone or with adenovirus and SV_{40}, there is significantly less biosynthesis of host-cell DNA than occurs in uninfected cells. It therefore seems likely that an active process blocks replication of host DNA rather than that its synthesis is merely not stimulated because synthesis of SV_{40} DNA is not permitted.

During the period before replication of SV_{40} DNA, the synthesis of one or more proteins is required for the enhanced production of adenovirus late proteins and thus the assembly of virions. Owing to its limited amount of genetic information, one may hypothesize that the protein is not a gene product of SV_{40} but rather that SV_{40} derepresses a host-cell protein which serves the required late adenovirus function. The hypothetical protein must be normally constitutive in KB cells and either constitutive in a small per cent of AGMK cells or present at a low level in many AGMK cells, thus permitting a small number of infectious adenovirus particles to be made under conditions of single infection. Alternatively, the genetic information necessary to synthesize the essential protein is present in the adenovirus genome, it is expressed in KB cells, but the function is restricted or the protein is inactivated in AGMK cells; infection with SV_{40} induces synthesis of a protein which may relieve the restriction or block the inactivation. This latter possibility could account for the finding that, with adenovirus alone, an increasing multiplicity of infection results in an increased yield of adenovirus. Thus, the presence of a greater number of functioning adenovirus genomes results in a greater opportunity for the postulated protein to participate in viral replication.

The intracellular interaction of SV_{40} and adenoviruses is not the sole example of biological and biochemical cooperation and conflict between animal viruses. For example, AAV are defective in all cells tested and their complete multiplication requires concomitant infection with an adenovirus (21, 29). However, while serving this helper function, the propagation of adenovirus is hindered (8, 30). The biochemical events responsible for the assistance and antagonism noted between viruses should elucidate some of the mechanisms which control the sequential transcription and translation of the genome in viral multiplication.

ACKNOWLEDGMENTS

This investigation was supported by Public Health Service research grants AI-03620 and 2-TI-AI-203 from the National Institute of Allergy and Infectious Diseases.

We thank Kathleen Coll and Joseph Higgs for their dedicated and excellent technical assistance.

LITERATURE CITED

1. Baserga, R. 1967. II. Autoradiographic methods, p. 45–110. *In* H. Busch (ed.), Methods in cancer research, vol. 1. Academic Press Inc., New York.
2. Baum, S. G., W. H. Weiss, and P. R. Reich. 1968. Studies on the mechanism of enhancement of adenovirus 7 infection in African green monkey cells by SV_{40}. Virology 34:373–376.
3. Bello, L. J., and H. S. Ginsberg. 1967. Inhibition of host protein synthesis in type 5 adenovirus-infected cells. J. Virol. 1:843–850.
4. Bello, L. J., and H. S. Ginsberg. 1969. Relationship between deoxyribonucleic acid-like ribonucleic acid synthesis and inhibition of host protein synthesis in type 5 adenovirus-infected KB cells. J. Virol. 3:106–113.
5. Black, P. H., E. M. Crawford, and L. V. Crawford. 1964. The purification of simian virus 40. Virology 24:381–387.
6. Burton, K. 1956. A study of the conditions and mechanisms of the diphenylamine reaction for the colorimetric estimation of deoxyribonucleic acid. Biochem. J. 62:315–323.
7. Carp, R. I., and R. S. Gilden. 1966. Comparison of replication cycles of SV_{40} in human diploid and African green monkey cells. Virology 28:150–162.
8. Casto, B. C., R. W. Atchison, and W. M. Hammon. 1967. Studies on the relationship between adeno-associated virus type I (AAV-I) and adenoviruses. I. Replication of AAV-I in certain cell cultures and its effect on helper adenovirus. Virology 32:52–59.
9. Crawford, L. V. and P. H. Black. 1964. The nucleic acid of SV_{40}. Virology 24:388–392.
10. Eagle, H. 1959. Amino acid metabolism in mammalian cell cultures. Science 130:432–437.
11. Feldman, L. H., J. S. Butel, and F. Rapp. 1966. Interaction of a simian papovavirus and adenovirus. I. Induction of adenovirus tumor antigen during abortive infection of simian cells. J. Bacteriol. 91:813–818.
12. Flanagan, J. F., and H. S. Ginsberg. 1962. Synthesis of virus-specific polymers in adenovirus-infected cells: effect of 5-fluorodeoxyuridine. J. Exp. Med. 116:141–157.
13. Gershon, D., L. Sachs, and E. Winocour. 1966. The induction of cellular DNA synthesis by simian virus 40 in contact-inhibited and X-irradiated cells. Proc. Nat. Acad. Sci. U.S.A. 56:918–925.
14. Gilead, Z., and H. S. Ginsberg. 1965. Characterization of a tumorlike antigen in type 12 and type 18 adenovirus infected cells. J. Bacteriol. 90:120–125.
15. Ginsberg, H. S., L. J. Bello, and A. J. Levine. 1967. Control of biosynthesis of host macromolecules in cells infected with adenovirus. p. 547–572. *In* J. S. Colter and W. Paranchych (ed.), Molecular biology of viruses. Academic Press Inc., New York.
16. Ginsberg, H. S., and M. J. Dixon. 1959. Deoxyribonucleic acid and protein alterations in HeLa cells infected with type 4 adenovirus. J. Exp. Med. 109:407–422.
17. Ginsberg, H. S., H. G. Pereira, R. C. Valentine, and W. C. Wilcox. 1966. A proposed terminology for the adenovirus antigens and virion morphological subunits. Virology 28:782–783.
18. Green, M. 1962. Studies on the viral biosynthesis of viral DNA. Cold Spring Harbor Symp. Quant. Biol. 27:219–235.
19. Hatanaka, M., and R. Dulbecco. 1966. Induction of DNA synthesis by SV_{40}. Proc. Nat. Acad. Sci. U.S.A. 56:736–740.
20. Hirt, B. 1966. Evidence for semi-conservative replication of circular polyoma DNA. Proc. Nat. Acad. Sci. U.S.A. 55:997–1004.

21. Hoggan, M. D., N. R., Blacklow, and W. P. Rowe. 1966. Studies of small DNA viruses found in various adenovirus preparations: physical, biological, and immunological characteristics. Proc. Nat. Acad. Sci. U.S.A. **55**:1467–1474.

22. Kit, S., R. A. de Torres, D. R. Dubbs, and M. C. Salvi. 1967. Induction of cellular deoxyribonucleic acid synthesis by simian virus 40. J. Viol. **1**:738–746.

23. Lawrence, W. C., and H. S. Ginsberg. 1967. Intracellular uncoating of type 5 adenovirus deoxyribonucleic acid. J. Virol. **1**:851–867.

24. Levine, A. J., and H. S. Ginsberg. 1967. Mechanism by which fiber antigen inhibits multiplication of type 5 adenovirus. J. Virol. **1**:747–757.

25. Malmgren, R. A., A. S. Rabson, P. G. Carney, and F. J. Paul. 1966. Immunofluorescence of green monkey kidney cells infected with adenovirus 12 and with adenovirus 12 plus simian virus 40. J. Bacteriol. **91**:262–265.

26. Mandell, J. D., and A. D. Hershey. 1960. A fractionating column for analysis of nucleic acids. Anal. Biochem. **1**:66–77.

27. Marmur, J. 1961. A procedure for the isolation of deoxyribonucleic acid from microorganisms. J. Mol. Biol. **3**:208–218.

28. O'Conor, G. T., A. S. Rabson, R. A. Malmgren, I. K. Berezesky, and F. J. Paul. 1965. Morphologic observations of green monkey kidney cells after single and double infection with adenovirus 12 and simian virus 40. J. Nat. Cancer Inst. **34**:679–693.

29. Parks, W. P., A. M. Casozza, J. Alcott, and J. L. Melnick. 1968. Adeno-associated satellite virus interference with the replication of its helper adenovirus. J. Exp. Med. **127**:91–108.

30. Philipson, L. 1961. Adenovirus assay by the fluorescent cell-counting procedure. Virology **15**:263–268.

31. Pope, J. H., and W. P. Rowe. 1964. Detection of specific antigen in SV40 transformed cells by immunofluorescence. J. Exp. Med. **120**:121–127.

32. Rabson, A. S., G. T. O'Conor, I. K. Berezesky, and F. J. Paul. 1964. Enhancement of adenovirus growth in African green monkey kidney cell cultures by SV40. Proc. Soc. Exp. Biol. Med. U.S.A. **116**:187–190.

33. Rapp, F., L. A. Feldman, and M. Mandel. 1966. Synthesis of virus deoxyribonucleic acid during abortive infection of simian cells by human adenovirus. J. Bacteriol. **92**:931–936.

34. Rapp, F., and M. Jerkofsky. 1967. Replication of PARA (defective SV40)-adenoviruses in simian cells. J. Gen. Virol. **1**:311–321.

35. Reich, P. R., S. G. Baum, J. A. Rose, W. P. Rowe, and S. M. Weissman. 1966. Nuclei acid homology studies of adenovirus type 7-SV40 interactions. Proc. Nat. Acad. Sci. U.S.A. **55**:336–341.

36. Russel, W. C., K. Hayashi, P. J. Sanderson, and H. G. Pereira. 1967. Adenovirus antigens—a study of their properties and sequential development in infection. J. Gen. Virol. **1**:495–507.

37. Sever, J. L. 1962. Application of a microtechnique to viral serological investigations. J. Immunol. **88**:320–329.

38. Sueoka, N., and T. Y. Cheng. 1962. Fractionation of nucleic acids with the methylated albumin column. J. Mol. Biol. **4**:161–172.

39. Thiel, J. F., and K. O. Smith. 1967. Fluorescent focus assay of viruses on cell monolayers in plastic petri dishes. Proc. Soc. Exp. Biol. Med. **125**:829–895.

40. Velicer, L. F., and H. S. Ginsberg. 1968. Cytoplasmic synthesis of type 5 adenovirus capsid proteins. Proc. Nat. Acad. Sci. U.S.A. **61**:1264–1271.

41. Vinograd, J., R. Bruner, R. Kent, and J. Weigle. 1963. Band centrifugation of macromolecules and viruses in self-generating density gradients. Proc. Nat. Acad. Sci. U.S.A. **49**:902–910.

42. Watson, J. D., and J. W. Littlefield. 1960. Some properties of DNA from shope papilloma virus. J. Mol. Biol. **2**:161–165.

Variation in Response of Syrian Hamster Lung Cells to Complete or Defective SV40 (PARA)[1]

M. Nachtigal and J. S. Butel

It was shown by the use of the immunofluorescence technique in 1964 that cells transformed by SV40 contained a new intranuclear antigen designated the tumor (T) antigen (1, 2). Later reports showed that newborn Syrian hamster lung cells appeared to transform following exposure to SV40 but did not develop detectable amounts of T antigen (3, 4).

A defective SV40 genome was subsequently demonstrated to be associated with a simian cell-adapted strain of adenovirus type 7 (5–7). The defective SV40 genome encased in an adenovirus capsid was named "PARA" (8) and was shown to carry the information for the synthesis of SV40 T antigen following either productive infection or transformation of cells (5–7, 9).

It was of interest to determine whether Syrian hamster lung cells responded to exposure to PARA the same as they did to SV40, particularly with respect to the synthesis of virus-specific antigens. This report shows that, in contrast to cultures exposed to parental SV40, the lung cells transformed by several different variants of PARA do contain detectable levels of SV40 T antigen.

Materials and Methods. Cells. Primary cultures of lung cells were prepared from a weanling male of the LSH inbred strain of Syrian hamsters obtained from Lakeview Hamster Colony, Newfield, New Jersey. The lungs were removed aseptically, minced, and trypsinized at 37° with a 0.25% (w/v) solution of trypsin.

Uninoculated and SV40-inoculated cultures were grown in Eagle's basal medium supplemented with 10% fetal bovine serum, 100 units/ml of penicillin, 100 μg/ml of streptomycin, 50 units/ml each of Mycostatin and Fungizone, and 0.075% sodium bicarbonate. Cells inoculated with PARA-adenovirus hybrid populations were grown in low calcium Eagle's minimal essential medium (10) supplemented as above. The low calcium medium was subsequently found not to be a requirement for the growth of the PARA-transformed cells.

Viruses. The Baylor reference strain of SV40 was used (11). It had been passed seven times in primary green monkey kidney (GMK) cells, plaque-purified in CV-1 cells, and then passed eight times in CV-1 cells. It had a titer of 1×10^7 plaque-forming units (PFU)/ml.

The L.L. strain of adenovirus 7, described elsewhere (7), was plaque-purified twice in GMK cells and clonal lines of virus were derived (12). The virus clones used in this study had been passed three times in GMK cells and were designated PARA (10nT)-adenovirus 7, PARA (39nT)-adenovirus 7, PARA (73nT)-adenovirus 7, PARA (1cT)-adenovirus 7 and PARA (2cT)-adenovirus 7. The titers of PARA in these stocks ranged from 0.5–5.0 $\times 10^5$ PFU/ml. PARA (1cT)-adenovirus 7 and PARA (2cT)-adenovirus 7 are unique in that they induce the synthesis of SV40 T antigen in the cytoplasm of cells (12, 13). PARA-adenovirus 16 was prepared by transcapsidation in a previous study (14), had undergone three passages in GMK cells, and had a PARA titer of 6×10^4 PFU/ml.

[1] Supported in part by Research Grant CA 04600 from the National Cancer Institute, National Institutes of Health, Bethesda, Maryland 20014.

TABLE I. Derivation of Cell Lines from Syrian Hamster Lung Cells Transformed *in Vitro* by SV40 and PARA-adenoviruses.[a]

Cell line	Transforming virus	MOI SV40 or PARA (PFU/cell)	Days pi		Morphology
			First passage	Second passage	
SHL-S	SV40	26	5	12	Fibroblastic
SHL-7 (10)	PARA (10nT)-Ad7	3.0	13	34	Fibroblastic
SHL-7 (39)	PARA (39nT)-Ad7	6.3	13	35	Fibroblastic
SHL-7 (73)	PARA (73nT)-Ad7	1.3	12	28	Fibroblastic
SHL-7 (1cT)	PARA (1cT)-Ad7	9.0	24	42	Fibroblastic
SHL-7 (2cT)	PARA (2cT)-Ad7	1.5	12	47	Fibroblastic
SHL-16	PARA-Ad16	0.06	5	14	Fibroblastic

[a] MOI = multiplicity of infection; pi = postinoculation.

Immunofluorescence techniques. The procedure used for the detection of SV40 and adenovirus T antigens has been described in detail (12). SV40 surface (S) antigen was detected on viable cells by the method of Tevethia *et al.* (15).

Transformation experiments. Two approaches were used to infect the cells in the transformation experiments. Method 1: Following the method of Duff and Rapp (16), secondary cultures of hamster lung cells were trypsinized and suspended in Eagle's medium, mixed with an equal volume of virus suspension, and shaken for 3 hr at 37°. At that time 0.4-ml aliquots of the suspension were distributed into 60-mm plastic petri dishes and 5 ml of complete growth medium were added to each dish. The cultures were incubated at 37° in an atmosphere of 5% CO_2 with fluid changes every 2–3 days. Method 2: Nonconfluent monolayers of fourth passage cultures of lung cells in 8-oz bottles were exposed to 1 ml of virus suspension. After a 3-hr adsorption period at 37° with intermittent shaking, 25 ml of growth medium were added/bottle.

Results. Growth characteristics of control and inoculated Syrian hamster lung cells. Control uninoculated lung cells (SHL) showed active proliferation for a period of approximately 2 months after explantation and could be passed weekly. After 2 months, the cells reached a stationary phase, could not be subcultured, and gradually died out.

No apparent cytopathic effects (CPE) were observed when the SHL cells were exposed to SV40 at a multiplicity of infection (MOI) of 26 PFU/cell (Table I). The exposed cells grew quickly and the culture medium rapidly became intensely acidified. At passage 16, the cell line (SHL-S) went into crisis, but recovered satisfactorily. The cells retained a fibroblastic morphology (Table I) and even at 7 months postinoculation (pi) did not exhibit any tendency to pile up.

All the cultures of SHL cells inoculated with different clonal lines of PARA-adenovirus hybrid populations at the MOI shown in Table I exhibited transitory adenovirus CPE. However, all the cultures recovered and were successfully subcultured at the intervals pi indicated in Table I. All the cells lines which were established from the PARA-infected cultures displayed a similar pattern of rapid and disorganized growth, intense acidification of the culture medium, and retention of a fibroblast-like morphology.

Presence of SV40 virus-specific antigens in transformed Syrian hamster lung cells. The PARA- and SV40-transformed hamster lung cell lines were tested by immunofluorescence for the presence of SV40 T and S antigens as well as adenovirus T antigen (Table II). The six cell lines derived from cultures transformed by different clonal lines of PARA all contained SV40 T antigen. As shown in Fig. 1, the intranuclear T antigen reaction observed with the PARA-transformed lung cells is typical of that seen in the majority of SV40-transformed cells. The fibroblastic morphology of the transformed lung cells is also apparent in Fig. 1.

TABLE II. Antigenic Analysis of Syrian Hamster Lung Cells Transformed *in Vitro* by PARA-adenoviruses and SV40.[a]

Cell line	SV40 T antigen		SV40 S antigen		Adeno T antigen	
	Passage	Result	Passage	Result	Passage	Result
SHL-7 (10)	4	+	7	+	11	0
SHL-7 (39)	3	+	7	+	8	+
SHL-7 (73)	4	+	12, 15	+	23	0
SHL-7 (1cT)	5	+ (cyto)	11	+	10	0
SHL-7 (2cT)	4	+	10, 12	+	14	0
SHL-16	10	+	11	+	16	+
SHL-S	5, 9, 13	0	9	0	Not done	

[a] + = presence of antigen, 0 = absence of antigen, cyto = cytoplasm.

In one cell line, SHL-7(1cT), the SV40 T antigen was spread diffusely throughout the cytoplasm with no reaction detected in the nucleus.

Repeated testings of the SV40-transformed cell line, SHL-S, with the same immunofluorescence reagents failed to reveal any SV40 T antigen positive cells (Table II). This observation is in agreement with that of previous reports (3, 4, 17).

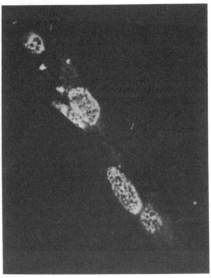

FIG. 1. Immunofluorescence detection of SV40 T antigen in Syrian hamster lung cells transformed by PARA (39nT)-adenovirus 7. Note fibroblastic morphology of the cells; ×400.

The transformed cell lines were first tested for the presence of SV40 S antigen between passages 7 and 12 (Table II). All the PARA-transformed lines contained this antigen at the cell membrane. However, S antigen was not detected in the lung cells exposed to SV40. This absence of S antigen correlates well with results obtained previously (18) with 3 of 6 SV40-transformed hamster lung cell lines.

Since adenovirions were present in all the stocks of PARA, the transformed cell lines were also assayed for the presence of adenovirus T antigen (Table II). Only the SHL-7(39) and SHL-16 cell lines contained detectable levels of adenovirus T antigen. However, animals bearing tumors induced by the SHL-7(73) and SHL-7(2cT) cells have yielded adenovirus T antibody, indicating that at least these two cell lines also contain adenovirus information.

Discussion. This paper demonstrates that PARA (defective SV40) can successfully transform Syrian hamster lung cells *in vitro*. Of particular interest is the observation that the lung cells transformed by PARA all contained detectable levels of SV40 T antigen. This is in contrast to cultures of lung cells exposed to parental SV40 which transformed but failed to synthesize SV40 T antigen. The response of SHL cells to complete and defective SV40 are compared in Table III. Four separate reports, originating from 3 different laboratories, have established that SHL cells consistently acquire an infinite life *in vitro* following exposure to SV40 but do not synthesize detectable amounts of T antigen.

130

| Virus | No. of lines | | No. of lines with SV40 antigens | | Ref. |
	Exposed	Transformed	T	S	
SV40	6	6	0	3	(3, 18)
SV40	1	1	0	ND[a]	(4)
SV40	1	1	0	ND	(17)
SV40	1	1	0	0	This report
PARA	6	6	6	6	This report

[a] ND = not done.

Some lines contain SV40 S antigen and others do not. In contrast, all 6 cultures exposed to variants of PARA in this study transformed and synthesized detectable levels of T and S antigens.

Although definitive evidence that SV40 is actually responsible for the observed transformation of the SHL-S cells is still lacking, the cells did undergo transformation following virus exposure, whereas companion control cultures did not. An increased growth potential was acquired by BHK21 cells after exposure to SV40 DNA in the absence of synthesis of T antigen (19), strengthening the possibility that a virus–cell relationship can occur which does not result in the synthesis of T antigen.

Several possible explanations are prompted by the difference observed in the response of lung cells to SV40 and PARA: (i) It has been shown that T antigen synthesis induced by PARA has a resistance to interferon more characteristic of adenoviruses than the comparative interferon sensitivity of T antigen induced by SV40 (20). This is probably due to the fact that a segment of adenovirus 7 DNA is covalently linked to the defective SV40 DNA in PARA (21, 22). Therefore, a superior capacity for interferon production could explain the variable response of Syrian hamster lung cells to T antigen synthesis induced by SV40 or PARA. In fact, organs containing phagocytic cells form interferon more rapidly than other tissues (23) and lung tissue contains a differentiated macrophagic type cell (24); (ii) we have shown by the use of lung cells from hybrid animals that a haploid chromosome complement from the Romanian hamster species alters the re-

sponse of the haploid Syrian hamster genome to SV40 such that T antigen is synthesized following transformation (25). Accordingly, the observed results might be a consequence of some contribution the cellular genome makes in determining the type of transformation, possibly at the level of regulation of transcription or translation of a persisting viral genome; (iii) the encasement of the defective SV40 genome in an adenocapsid and the presence of complete adenovirions in the PARA inocula may have, in some way, altered adsorption, penetration, uncoating, or subsequent events following virus inoculation; (iv) while the PARA genome probably does persist in the transformed cultures, it is possible that, in contrast, SV40 actually mediated the transformation observed in the SHL-S cells, but no longer persists. Evidence currently available does not allow us to distinguish between the possible explanations outlined above.

This study confirms previous observations [(26), Richardson and Butel, in preparation] that SV40 T antigen can be localized in the cytoplasm of transformed cells. It also demonstrates the variable response that can be observed with differentiated host cells with respect to the expression of virus-specific antigens after exposure to viruses containing similar genetic information. This observation is pertinent in view of attempts to detect virus-specific antigens as an approach to demonstrating a viral etiology of human tumors.

Summary. Adult Syrian hamster lung cells were exposed to six clonal lines of PARA (defective SV40) as well as to parental SV40. All the exposed cultures transformed. SV40

T and S antigens were synthesized in all the cells transformed by PARA, but could not be detected in the culture which transformed following exposure to SV40.

1. Pope, J. H., and Rowe, W. P., J. Exp. Med. 120, 121 (1964).
2. Rapp, F., Butel, J. S., and Melnick, J. L., Proc. Soc. Exp. Biol. Med. 116, 1131 (1964).
3. Diamandopoulos, G. T., and Enders, J. F., Proc Nat. Acad. Sci. U.S.A. 54, 1092 (1965).
4. Van der Noordaa, J., and Enders, J. F., Proc. Soc. Exp. Biol. Med. 122, 1144 (1966).
5. Huebner, R. J., Chanock, R. M., Rubin, B. A., and Casey, M. J., Proc. Nat. Acad. Sci. U.S.A. 52, 1333 (1964).
6. Rowe, W. P., and Baum, S. G., Proc. Nat. Acad. Sci. U.S.A. 52, 1340 (1964).
7. Rapp, F., Melnick, J. L., Butel, J. S., and Kitahara, T., Proc. Nat. Acad. Sci. U.S.A. 52, 1348 (1964).
8. Rapp, F., Butel, J. S., and Melnick, J. L., Proc. Nat. Acad. Sci. U.S.A. 54, 717 (1965).
9. Black, P. H., and Todaro, G. J., Proc. Nat. Acad. Sci. U.S.A. 54, 374 (1965).
10. Freeman, A. E., Calisher, C. H., Price, P. J., Turner, H. C., and Huebner, R. J., Proc. Soc. Exp. Biol. Med. 122, 835 (1966).
11. Rapp, F., Butel, J. S., Feldman, L. A., Kitahara, T., and Melnick, J. L., J. Exp. Med. 121, 935 (1965).
12. Rapp, F., Pauluzzi, S., and Butel, J. S., J. Virol. 4, 626 (1969).
13. Butel, J. S., Guentzel, M. J., and Rapp, F., J. Virol. 4, 632 (1969).
14. Rapp, F., Jerkofsky, M., Melnick, J. L., and Levy, B., J. Exp. Med. 127, 77 (1968).
15. Tevethia, S. S., Katz, M., and Rapp, F., Proc. Soc. Exp. Biol. Med. 119, 896 (1965).
16. Duff, R., and Rapp, F., J. Virol. 5, 568 (1970).
17. Sahnazarov, N., Graffe, L. H., Nachtigal, M., and Ionescu-Homoriceanu, S., Rev. Roum. Inframi crobiol. 7, 79 (1970).
18. Diamandopoulos, G. T., Tevethia, S. S., Rapp, F., and Enders, J. F., Virology 34, 331 (1968).
19. Black, P. H., and Rowe, W. P., Proc. Nat. Acad. Sci. U.S.A. 54, 1126 (1965).
20. Oxman, M. N., Rowe, W. P., and Black, P. H., Proc. Nat. Acad. Sci. U.S.A. 57, 941 (1967).
21. Baum, S. G., Reich, P. R., Hybner, C. J., Rowe, W. P., and Weissman, S. M., Proc. Nat. Acad. Sci. U.S.A. 56, 1509 (1966).
22. Levin, M. J., Black, P. H., Coghill, S. L., Dixon, C. B., and Henry, P. H., J. Virol. 4, 704 (1969).
23. Kono, Y., and Ho, M., Virology 25, 162 (1965).
24. Bowden, D. H., Adamson, I. Y. R., Grantham, G., and Wyatt, J. P., Arch. Pathol. 88, 540 (1968).
25. Nachtigal, M., Sahnazarov, N., Butel, J. S., and Melnick, J. L., Bacteriol. Proc. 1970, 186.
26. Duff, R., Rapp, F., and Butel, J. S., Virology 42, 273 (1970).

Requirement for Cell Replication after SV40 Infection for a Structural Change of the Cell Surface Membrane

HANNAH BEN-BASSAT, MICHAEL INBAR, AND LEO SACHS

INTRODUCTION

Studies with the carbohydrate-binding protein concanavalin A (Con. A), which binds to sites on the cell surface membrane, have shown a difference in the structure of the surface membrane between normal and transformed cells. About 85% of the binding sites for this protein that are exposed on the surface membrane of transformed cells are in a cryptic form on normal cells (Inbar and Sachs, 1969a). Owing to this exposure of sites on the surface, transformed cells can be agglutinated by Con. A, whereas normal and 3T3 cells are not agglutinated under the same conditions (Inbar and Sachs, 1969b). Infection of normal cells with polyoma virus and of 3T3 cells with simian virus 40 (SV40) results in a gain of agglutinability several days after infection of multiplying cultures (Inbar and Sachs, 1969b). This suggested that the change in the structure of the surface membrane after virus infection that results in agglutinability, which was also found in abortively trans- formed cells (Inbar and Sachs, 1969b), may require cell replication. The present experiments with 3T3 cells and SV40 were undertaken (1) to obtain direct evidence for such a requirement for cell replication, (2) to determine the number of cell generations required, and (3) to determine whether the loss of agglutinability in abortively trans- formed cells also requires cell replication.

MATERIALS AND METHODS

Cell cultures. Cells of the untransformed line 3T3 were used between the 5th and 8th subculture after receiving the cells from Dr. H. Green. A line of SV40 transformed 3T3 cells was also received from Dr. H. Green. The cells were cultured in Eagle's medium with a 4-fold concentration of amino acids and vitamins (EM) with 10% calf serum in 50 mm plastic (Falcon Co.) petri dishes. Cells were routinely passaged in a 0.25% trypsin (1:300) solution, and for the ex- periments on agglutinability after subcul- turing, with a 0.02% EDTA solution (Inbar and Sachs, 1969b).

Infection with SV40. The strain 776 of SV40 was used. Virus stocks were obtained after infection of the cell line BS-C-1 with a low input (Uchida *et al.*, 1966), not more than 0.1 plaque forming unit (PFU) per cell, and the stocks were harvested when a complete cytopathic effect was observed. 3T3 cells were infected with 10 PFU of SV40 per cell, one day after the cells were seeded in 50-mm petri dishes. After 2 hours for virus absorption, the cells were washed once with phosphate-buffered saline (PBS), and new EM with 10% calf serum was added. Control cultures were treated with an equal amount of a sonicated extract of uninfected BS-C-1 cells.

Agglutination assay with concanavalin A (Con. A). As in previous experiments (Inbar and Sachs, 1969a,b) the protein was prepared from jackbean meal (Sigma Chemical Co.) by 2 crystallizations, and stored as a solution in saturated NaCl at room temperature. For the agglutination assay, (Inbar and Sachs, 1969b) cells were washed 2 or 3 times with Ca- and Mg-free PBS and removed from the petri dish with a solution of 0.02% EDTA in 8 g of NaCl, 0.2 g of KCl, 1.15 g of Na_2HPO_4, and 0.2 g of KH_2PO_4 per 1000 ml of distilled water. The suspended cells were washed 3 times with Ca- and Mg-free PBS, and then diluted in Ca- and Mg-free PBS at a concentration of 0.5 to 1 × 10^6 cells per milliliter. To test for agglutination, 0.5 ml of Con. A diluted in distilled water or Ca- and Mg-free PBS was mixed with 0.5 ml of cell suspension in a 35 mm petri dish (Falcon Co.) at a final concentration of 500 μg Con. A per milliliter. The density and size of aggregates was scored in a scale from − to ++++ after 30 min incubation at room temperature.

Detection of SV40 nuclear tumor (T) antigen. The immunofluorescence test for the T antigen induced by SV40 was made as in previous experiments (Gershon *et al.*, 1966), with fluorescein-conjugated anti-SV40 hamster serum by the direct method after acetone fixing. The percent of cells with T antigen was calculated from a count of 500 cells.

Transformation assay. Infected cells were seeded for cloning 1 day after virus infection at 100 or 1000 cells per 50 mm petri dish, and the cells were stained with Giemsa at 18 days after seeding. The cloning efficiency was determined from plates seeded at 100 cells. The number of transformed colonies was determined by counting colonies that grew over the monolayer in plates seeded at 1000 cells. The percent transformed colonies is given as a percent of the total number of colonies.

RESULTS

Correlation between agglutinability and Cell Replication after Virus Infection

In order to determine the effect of cell replication after virus infection on agglutinability, 3T3 cells were seeded at 4 different seeding levels. Agglutinability by Con. A was tested daily after virus infection. The 4 seeding levels were chosen to give either different amounts or almost no cell multiplication at various times before the cultures became confluent (Table 1). At 6 days after virus infection, the average number of cell generations in the 4 sets of cultures were 4.18, 2.30, 1.04, and 0.15 (Table 2). The cultures which showed only 0.15 cell generations at 6 days will be referred to as nonmultiplying cultures. The results indi-

TABLE 1

TOTAL NUMBER OF CELLS AND CELL DENSITY IN INFECTED CULTURES AT DIFFERENT SEEDING LEVELS

Seeding level (No. of cells × 10^{-5})	Days after virus infection			
	0^a	2	4	6
	Total number of cells × 10^{-5}			
2	1.4	6.0	18.0	26.5
5	4.8	9.8	23.5	25.0
12	12.0	15.0	22.0	25.0
20	20.0	19.4	20.0	23.0
	Cell density per cm^2 × 10^{-5}			
2	0.07	0.30	0.90	1.32
5	0.24	0.49	1.17	1.25
12	0.60	0.75	1.10	1.25
20	1.00	0.87	1.00	1.15

^{a} 0 time = one day after seeding, when cells were infected with SV40.

134

TABLE 2

Percent of Cells with T Antigen and Percent Transformed Colonies in Cultures Seeded at Different Seeding Levels

Seeding level. (No. of cells $\times 10^{-5}$)	Average number of cell generations at 6 days after virus infection	Days after virus infection			% transformed colonies[a]
		2	4	6	
		% cells with T antigen			
2	4.18	13	31	34	0.7
5	2.30	22	30	33	1.2
12	1.04	23	24	27	0.6
20	0.15	3	5	3	0.5

[a] The percent transformed colonies was determined from cells seeded for cloning at 1 day after virus infection.

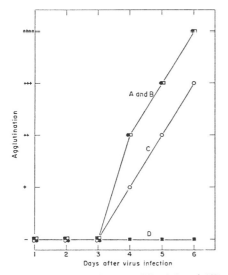

Fig. 1. Agglutinability of SV40-infected 3T3 cells seeded at 2×10^5 (A), 5×10^5 (B), 12×10^5 (C), and 20×10^5 (D) cells per petri dish. The cells were infected 1 day after seeding.

cate (Fig. 1) that agglutination by Con. A was found only in the multiplying cultures. These cultures first started to agglutinate at day 4 after virus infection, and the degree of agglutinability increased between 4 and 6 days. In cultures with the maximum degree

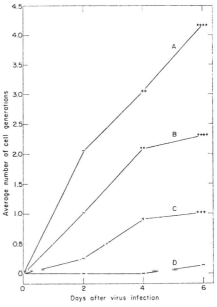

Fig. 2. Average number of cell generations and agglutinability of SV40 infected 3T3 cells. The seeding levels for A, B, C, and D are the same as those given in the legend to Fig. 1.

of agglutination at 6 days, about 50% of cells had formed aggregates containing about 30–100 cells each. Uninfected 3T3 cells were not agglutinated by Con. A at any of the seeding levels tested.

When the multiplying cultures started to agglutinate at 4 days after virus infection, the cultures seeded at different seeding levels had reached 1 to 3 cell generations (Fig. 2) and they all had a cell density of about 10^5 cells per cm^2 (Table 1). The lack of agglutinability in cultures which had undergone 1 or 2 cell generations at 2 days (Fig. 2), but had at this time reached a density of only 5 or 3×10^4 cells per cm^2 (Table 1) indicates that the gain of agglutinability requires at least 1 cell generation and a density of about 10^5 cells per cm^2. The nonmultiplying cultures in which the cells did not undergo at least 1 cell generation showed no gain of agglutinability even though they reached a density of about 10^5 cells per cm^2 (Table 1).

135

Experiments with a line of SV40 transformed 3T3 cells have indicated, that cultures seeded at 2×10^5 or 2×10^6 cells per plate were not agglutinated by Con. A at 1 or 2 days after seeding, but that at both seeding levels these transformed cells were agglutinated $(+++)$ at 3 days.

Percent of Cells with T Antigen and Percent Transformed Colonies

The results shown in Table 2 indicate that all the multiplying cultures contained about 30% cells with T antigen whereas the nonmultiplying cultures contained only about 3% cells with T antigen. The percent of cells with T antigen in the multiplying cultures is of about the same order of magnitude as the 50% of cells that formed aggregates at 6 days after virus infection. The aggregates, collected with a micropipette, were dissociated with 10^{-1} M α-methyl-D-glucopyranoside (Inbar and Sachs, 1969b), and the cells were then incubated overnight on coverslips. About 90% of these cells contained T antigen. As in previous experiments (Inbar and Sachs, 1969b), the percent of cells agglutinated is much higher than the about 1% cells that formed transformed colonies (Table 2). The present results thus also indicate that agglutination occurred between cells with abortive transformation.

Loss of Agglutinability after Cell Replication

In order to determine whether the loss of agglutinability in cells with abortive transformation requires cell replication, SV40 infected 3T3 cells seeded at 5×10^5 cells per petri dish were subcultured at 6 days after virus infection when the cultures had reached the maximum degree of agglutination. The subcultures were seeded at 2×10^5 cells per plate to give multiplying cultures, and at 2×10^6 cells per plate to give nonmultiplying cultures. The results of agglutination assays indicate (Table 3 and Fig. 3) that the multiplying cultures had completely lost agglutinability at 3 days after subculturing, at which time they had undergone 1.7 cell generations (Fig. 3). However, the nonmultiplying cultures with an average of 0.12 cell generation at 3 days after subculturing did not show this loss of agglutinability. Both the multiplying and the nonmultiplying subcultures showed a similar percent of cells with T antigen (Table 3).

TABLE 3

AGGLUTINATION AND PERCENT OF CELLS WITH T ANTIGEN AFTER SUBCULTURE OF INFECTED CELLS

	Nonmultiplying culture. Days after subculture			Multiplying culture. Days after subculture		
	1	2	3	1	2	3
Total number of cells $\times 10^{-5}$	17.0	19.0	19.0	2.5	6.5	8.5
Agglutination	+++	+++	+++	+++	+	—
% cells with T antigen	15	13	14	11	11	12

" Cells were subcultured at 6 days after virus infection, at which time the cultures had an agglutinability of $++++$ and 20% cells with T antigen.

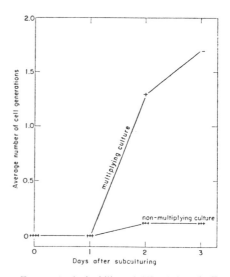

FIG. 3. Agglutinability of SV40 infected 3T3 cells after subculturing as multiplying and non-multiplying cultures.

DISCUSSION

The present results have indicated that the change in the structure of the cell surface membrane that results in a gain of agglutinability by Con. A after SV40 infection of 3T3 cells requires at least 1 cell generation and a density of about 10^5 cells per cm.[2] It will be of interest to determine whether the requirement for cell density involves a requirement for cell to cell contacts and/or a threshold amount of some substance produced by the cells. Previous results have indicated a requirement for cell replication for cell transformation induced by carcinogenic hydrocarbons (Berwald and Sachs, 1965), X-irradiation (Borek and Sachs, 1966, 1967; Sachs, 1966) and SV40 (Todaro and Green, 1966); and that 1 cell generation is required to fix transformation by SV40 (Todaro and Green, 1966) and 2 cell generations are required to fix transformation by X-irradiation (Borek and Sachs, 1968). Agglutinability by Con. A has been found with cells transformed by chemical carcinogens, X-irradiation, SV40 and other agents (Inbar and Sachs, 1969b). The requirement for the change in the structure of the surface membrane thus appears to be associated with the requirement for cell transformation.

The about 50% cells agglutinated after SV40 infection was of about the same order of magnitude as the percent of cells with T antigen, and this antigen was found in about 90% of the agglutinated cells. The frequency of agglutinated cells was much higher than the about 1% cells that were hereditarily transformed. It has previously been observed, that a temporary change of some cellular properties can be found after infection with polyoma virus in a much higher percent of cells than those that are hereditarily transformed (Medina and Sachs, 1961; Stoker, 1968) a phenomenon that has been called abortive transformation (Stoker, 1968). The present and previous results (Inbar and Sachs, 1969b), thus indicate that abortive transformation can produce the same change in the structure of the surface membrane as hereditary transformation. The results further indicate, that the loss of this change in structure in abortively transformed cells requires cell replication. It will be of interest to determine whether the loss of agglutinability by Con. A in variants from polyoma-transformed cells with a reversion of properties of transformed cells (Inbar et al., 1969; Rabinowitz and Sachs, 1969) requires cell replication.

A difference in the structure of the surface membrane between untransformed and transformed cells has also been suggested from studies with a wheat germ agglutinin (Burger, 1969), a glycoprotein that binds to different carbohydrates than Con. A. It has also been found that there is a gain of agglutinability by this wheat germ agglutinin in 3T3 cells abortively transformed by SV40 (Burger, Inbar, and Sachs, to be published).

ACKNOWLEDGMENTS

This study was supported by contract No. 69-2014 within the Special Virus-Cancer Program of the National Cancer Institute, National Institutes of Health, U.S. Public Health Service.

We are indebted to Mrs. Mechtild Ebenhoh and Miss Ilana Kiwiti for skillful technical assistance.

REFERENCES

BERWALD, Y., and SACHS, L. (1965). In vitro transformation of normal cells to tumor cells by carcinogenic hydrocarbons. J. Natl. Cancer Inst. 35, 641–661.

BOREK, C., and SACHS, L. (1966). In vitro cell transformation by X-irradiation. Nature 210, 276–278.

BOREK, C., and SACHS, L. (1967). Cell susceptibility to transformation by X-irradiation and fixation of the transformed state. Proc. Natl. Acad. Sci. U.S. 57, 1522–1527.

BOREK, C., and SACHS, L. (1968). The number of cell generations required to fix the transformed state in X-ray induced transformation. Proc. Natl. Acad. Sci. U.S. 59, 83–85.

BURGER, M. M. (1969). A difference in the architecture of the surface membrane of normal and virally transformed cells. Proc. Natl. Acad. Sci. U.S. 62, 994–1001.

GERSHON, D., SACHS, L., and WINOCOUR, E. (1966). The induction of cellular DNA synthesis by simian virus 40 in contact inhibited and in X-irradiated cells. Proc. Natl. Acad. Sci. U.S. 56, 918–925.

INBAR, M., and SACHS, L. (1969a). Structural differences in sites on the surface membrane of normal and transformed cells. *Nature* **223**, 710-712.

INBAR, M., and SACHS, L. (1969b). Interaction of the carbohydrate-binding protein concanavalin A with normal and transformed cells. *Proc. Natl. Acad. Sci. U.S.* **63**, 1418-1425.

INBAR, M., RABINOWITZ, Z., and SACHS, L. (1969). The formation of variants with a reversion of properties of transformed cells. III. Reversion of the structure of the cell surface membrane. *Intern. J. Cancer* **4**, 690-696.

MEDINA, D., and SACHS, L. (1961). Cell-virus interaction with the polyoma virus. III. The induction of cell transformation and malignancy *in vitro*, *Brit. J. Cancer* **15**, 885-904.

RABINOWITZ, Z., and SACHS, L. (1969). The formation of variants with a reversion of properties of transformed cells. IV. Loss of detectable polyoma transplantation antigen. *Virology* in press.

SACHS, L. (1966). An analysis of the mechanism of carcinogenesis by polyoma virus, hydrocarbons, and X-irradiation. *In* "Molekulare Biologie des malignen Wachstums" pp. 242-255. Springer, New York.

STOKER, M. (1968). Abortive transformation by polyoma virus. *Nature* **218**, 234-238.

SUMMER, J. B., and HOWELL, S. F. (1936). The identification of the hemagglutinin of the jackbean with concanavalin A. *J. Bacteriol.* **32**, 227-237.

TODARO, G. J., and GREEN, H. (1966). Cell growth and the initiation of transformation by SV40. *Proc. Natl. Acad Sci. U.S.* **55**, 302-308.

UCHIDA, S., WATANABE, S., and KATO, M. (1966). Incomplete growth of simian virus 40 in African green monkey culture induced by serial undiluted passages. *Virology* **28**, 135-141.

138

Encapsidation of Free Host DNA by Simian Virus 40: A Simian Virus 40 Pseudovirus

David M. Trilling
David Axelrod

The phenomenon of encapsidation of host DNA has been shown to exist in polyoma virus (1, 2). Simian virus 40 (2), another member of the papovavirus group, has not been shown to contain within the viral capsid host cell DNA unlinked to viral DNA. Aloni et al. have presented evidence suggesting that the SV40 genome may contain host DNA sequences as part of the viral DNA (3). We now report that a portion of the host DNA becomes encapsidated and that this portion has a lower molecular weight than virus DNA has. Plaque purified, SV40 small plaque (SP) was grown on Vero cells, a continuous green monkey cell line. During the purification of virus passed in Vero cells, two bands became apparent in CsCl equilibrium density centrifugation. The upper virus band, which has a lower density in CsCl, was found to contain host DNA and DNA species of a lower molecular weight than that present in the lower virus band. Additional experiments, in which cell DNA was labeled with [^{32}P]orthophosphate prior to infection, have demonstrated encapsidation of linear host DNA with a sedimentation value of 15.

The SV40 SP was separated from disrupted Vero cells and culture medium by zone sedimentation on to a CsCl cushion (1.40 g/cm^3) followed by two cycles of CsCl equilibrium density centrifugation. At these concentrations CsCl dissociates DNA-protein complexes and leaves intact complete virus stripped of extracapsid DNA. Further, in certain experiments, the virus was treated with pancreatic deoxyribonuclease and ribonuclease after CsCl centrifugation. Virus DNA for immobilization on filters was extracted by lysing the virus in 1 percent SDS at 50°C. Then CsCl was added to precipitate the SDS, the precipitate was removed by centrifugation, and the double-stranded circular DNA-I was separated by equilibrium density centrifugation in CsCl containing ethidium bromide (4). The dye was removed by treatment with Dowex-50, and the CsCl was removed by Sephadex G-100 gel filtration. Host DNA was prepared by conventional methods (5). DNA-DNA hybridization was performed basically as described by Denhardt (6) but on a microscale (7). The SV40 DNA-I to be immobilized was first heated at 100°C for 15 minutes in SSC (2) to break the circle, denatured with alkali, rapidly diluted in 4 × SSC, neutralized and finally poured through a nitrocellulose membrane filter, 5.0 cm in diameter. Host cell DNA was similarly treated, but the heating step was omitted. Filters containing DNA and blank control filters, 7 mm in diameter, were cut from the large filters and given preliminary incubation at 68°C under Denhardt's conditions. After this incubation period, samples of fragmented (sheared in a Biosonik II to approximately 400,000 daltons), heat-denatured, and labeled DNA to be tested were introduced into test tubes (10 by 25 mm) with the filters. The final reaction mixture (0.25 ml) contained $1.0M$ NaCl, $0.004M$ TES, pH 7.5, and PM (2).

Virions containing host DNA, termed SV40 pseudovirions, were observed after passage of plaque-purified SV40 SP in Vero cells (passage numbers 165 to 170) at an input multiplicity of 1 to 10 plaque-forming units per cell. After CsCl equilibrium centrifugation, the virus was distributed into two bands. Although the appearance of the upper band resembled that of defective virus, the band contained host DNA and noncircular DNA. The appearance of DNA in a form other than the double-stranded circle distinguishes these particles from the defective particles described by Yoshiike (8).

Vero cells were grown in a half-gallon roller bottle in Eagle's medium with 10 percent fetal bovine serum (FBS). At confluency, the cells were infected, at an input multiplicity of 1, with SV40 SP passed two times in Vero cells. After a 2-hour adsorption period, fresh medium with 5 percent FBS was added. Twenty-four hours after infection, the medium was removed and fresh medium (100 ml) with 2 percent FBS and 250 μc of [³H]thymidine (14 c/mmole) was added. The cells and culture medium were harvested 72 hours later and the virus was purified as described earlier (Fig. 1). The virus shows a peak at 1.348 g/cm³ with a shoulder at 1.341 g/cm³. Two bands are clearly apparent on examination of the tube but are only partially resolved on tube puncture and drop collection. The virus particles in both pools (pool 1, fractions 24 to 28; pool 2, fractions 30 to 36) are indistinguishable by negative staining in the electron microscope and are similar in size. As was determined in the Spinco Model E ultracentrifuge the sedimentation coefficient ($s^0_{20,w}$) value of pool 1 is 211; that of pool 2 was 224. However, differences are readily apparent when virus pools are lysed in $0.1N$ NaOH and sedimented in an alkaline sucrose gradient, with an SV40 SP marker made on low-passage Vero cells (passage 40) at an input multiplicity of 0.01 (Fig. 2).

The alkaline sedimentation profile of the DNA from pool 1 closely resembles that of the DNA from the marker virus. Since the double-stranded, closed, circular DNA of the mature virus sediments at $53S$ under alkaline conditions, this DNA form can be readily distinguished from linear and nicked, circular DNA forms that have the same molecular weight but have components sedimenting at 18 and $16S$ under alkaline conditions (9). In pool 1, 75 percent of the DNA is in the closed circular form. However, in pool 2, only 50 percent of the DNA is in the closed circular form. The remaining 50 percent is not only in single circles and linear DNA but in even shorter pieces, that is $6S$ or smaller, sedimenting close to the meniscus. The profile of pool 2 further indicates that the DNA in the $53S$ and $18S$ regions has a slightly lower molecular weight than the DNA in the marker virus has. The DNA from pool 2 in these two regions is skewed toward the slower sedimenting side of the 53S and 18S peaks of the DNA from the marker virus. The lower molecular weights of the DNA's in virus particles of pool 2 account for its lower density, relative to pool 1. The lower molecular weight of the DNA in a virus particle decreases the DNA-protein ratio which has the effect of lowering the density of the whole particle.

Hybridization of the DNA from the two pools with the host DNA shows that, whereas 3.3 percent from pool 1 hybridizes with host DNA, 13.0 percent from pool 2 hybridizes with host DNA. Since specific activities were approximately equal, the host DNA content of pool 2 is at least four times that of pool 1. In a subsequent experiment, hybridization was performed with material recovered from an alkaline sucrose gradient (as in Fig. 1). From the 18S region of pool 2, 16.8 percent of the DNA hybridized with the host DNA, whereas from the 18S region of pool 1 only 3.0 percent of the DNA hybridized with the host. The DNA from the 53S regions of pools 1 and 2 reacted only with viral DNA. No reaction with host DNA was detected.

To delineate the encapsidation of host DNA by the SV40 virus, Vero cells were grown in three half-gallon roller bottles in phosphate-free Eagle's medium (150 ml) with 3 percent normal FBS, 6 percent FBS dialyzed against 0.15M NaCl, and 2.5 mc of carrier-free [^{32}P]orthophosphate. When the cells were confluent, they were washed with complete medium and then exposed to complete medium with 10 percent normal FBS. One day later, the cells were infected at a multiplicity of 5 with SV40 SP that had been passed twice in Vero cells. After a 2-hour adsorption period, fresh complete medium with 2 percent FBS was added. At 96 hours, the cells and culture medium were harvested, and the virus was purified as described, except that an additional CsCl equilibrium centrifugation was used. The two discrete bands were collected separately with a curved needle and syringe rather than by the drop method. The upper band (1.341 g/cm^3) and the lower band (1.348 g/cm^3) were dialyzed and treated with pancreatic deoxyribonuclease and ribonuclease as described in Table 1. A fraction of each band was lysed in NaOH, neutralized with HCl, sonicated, denatured by heat, and then tested by hybridization against Vero and SV40 DNA's. The virus from the upper band is rich in host DNA, whereas the virus from the lower band has mainly viral DNA (Table 1). On the basis of a comparison of these results with the extents of reaction in control experiments (Table 1, numbers 5 and 8), the ^{32}P from the upper band is primarily in host DNA. Because of the size of host DNA and presence of unique sequences, host DNA reacts to a lesser extent than viral DNA.

The virus from the upper and lower bands was lysed in NaOH, and the DNA was analyzed in alkaline sucrose density gradients (Fig. 3). The [^{3}H]-thymidine-labeled DNA from marker virus, grown on Vero cells with seed passed one time in Vero cells, had two peaks, 53S and 18S, in a 1:1 ratio. The 53S peak represents the double-stranded intact circle of the mature virus; the 18S peak represents the single strands of linear and nicked, circular DNA's. The upper band virus harvested from cells previously labeled with ^{32}P yielded 53S and 18S components in a ratio of 1 to 3.4, whereas the lower band virus yielded 53S and 18S components in a ratio of 1 to 0.36.

This difference in ratios is a reflection of the differing content of host

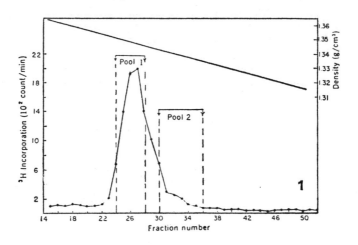

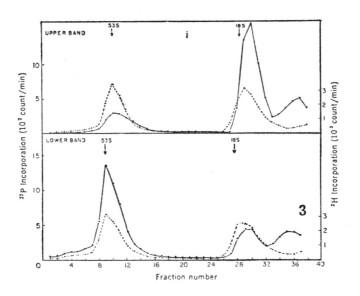

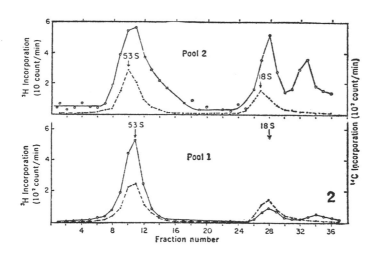

Fig. 1. Purification of SV40 from Vero cells, labeled with
[³H]thymidine after infection, in a second CsCl density gradient in the angle-head Spinco No. 65 rotor (35,000 rev/min for
18 hours). Fractions were collected from the bottom of the
centrifuge tube, and the radioactive material in a sample of
each fraction was determined by precipitating with trichloroacetic acid, collecting on a membrane filter, and counting in a
scintillation counter.   Fig. 2. Band sedimentation in alkaline
sucrose gradients of [³H]thymidine-labeled pools 1 and 2 with
[¹⁴C]thymidine-labeled marker virus. Virus samples were lysed
in 0.1N NaOH and sedimented through a sucrose gradient (5
to 20 percent) in 0.30M NaOH, 0.70M NaCl, 0.01M tris-HCl,
pH 7.5, 0.001M EDTA at 40,000 rev/min for 4 hours in the
Spinco SW 65 rotor. Fractions were collected from the bottom
of the tube, and each fraction was precipitated with trichloroacetic acid, collected on a membrane filter, dried, and counted.
Fig. 3. Band sedimentation in alkaline sucrose gradients of
upper and lower band virus prepared from ³²P-labeled cells
with [³H]thymidine–labeled marker virus. Virus samples, lysed
in NaOH, were sedimented through an alkaline sucrose gradient
(5 to 20 percent) as described for Fig. 2.

DNA in the upper and lower bands
(Table 1). To use hybridization to
identify the slower sedimenting component at 18S as the host DNA, sedimentation in the alkaline sucrose gradients was repeated in the absence of
marker. The [³²P]DNA's from the 53S
region and from the 18S region were
collected, dialyzed, sonicated, denatured with heat, and then tested against
Vero and SV40 DNA's. The ³²P from
the 53S regions from the upper and
lower bands of virus was bound ef-
ficiently to the SV40 DNA filter but
not at all to the host DNA filter (Table
2). The ³²P from the 18S regions reacted with both the host and viral
DNA filters. However, the extent of
reaction with the host filter from upper
band is threefold greater than with

143

Table 1. Hybridization of DNA from upper and lower bands of SV40 with SV40 and Vero cell DNA's. DNA on Vero filter, 10 μg; on SV40 filter, 0.6 μg. Prior to DNA extraction, virus was treated with pancreatic deoxyribonuclease (20 μg/ml) and pancreatic ribonuclease (75 μg/ml) for 1 hour at 25°C in phosphate-buffered saline with 0.004M MgCl$_2$.

Reaction No.	DNA		Amounts incubated (count/min)	Specifically bound (% of input)
	On filter	Source in solution		
1	SV40	Upper band	7500 (^{32}P)	16.2
2	Vero*	Upper band	7500 (^{32}P)	17.9
3	SV40	Lower band	9100 (^{32}P)	26.4
4	Vero	Lower band	9100 (^{32}P)	5.3
5	SV40	SV40 DNA-I	2800 (^{14}C, 0.12 μg)	61.9
6	Vero	SV40 DNA-I	2800 (^{14}C, 0.12 μg)	0.76
7	SV40	Vero DNA	28000 (^{14}C, 1.4 μg)	0.03
8	Vero	Vero DNA	28000 (^{14}C, 1.4 μg)	24.1

* As performed, the DNA-DNA hybridization tests between Vero cell DNA and sample measure only the repetitive nucleotide sequences, not the unique sequences. Single copies of SV40 DNA in the host DNA would not have been detected (11).

Table 2. DNA-DNA hybridization tests between Vero cell DNA and two components of ^{32}P-labeled SV40 isolated by band sedimentation in alkaline sucrose gradients. DNA on Vero filter, 10 μg; on SV40 filter, 0.6 μg.

Reaction No.	DNA		^{32}P incubated (count/min)	Radioactivity	
	On filter	In solution		Bound to filter (count/min)	% of input
	Upper band virus				
1	SV40	53S	960	616	64.2
	None			1	0.1
2	Vero*	53S	960	0	0
	None			0	0
3	SV40	18S	2300	219	9.5
	None			1	< 0.1
4	Vero	18S	2300	626	27.2
	None			2	< 0.1
	Lower band virus				
5	SV40	53S	1675	871	52.0
	None			0	0
6	Vero	53S	1675	1	< 0.1
	None			0	0
7	SV40	18S	920	237	25.8
	None			1	0.1
8	Vero	18S	920	186	20.2
	None			0	0

* See footnote to Table 1.

145

the viral filter. Comparison of these results with the extents of reaction in control experiments (Table 1, numbers 5 and 8) indicates that the ^{32}P in the 18S region of the upper band virus is primarily in host DNA, not in viral DNA. The appearance of ^{32}P in viral DNA in the 53S region, the intact double-stranded circle, is presumably a result of either complete breakdown and resynthesis of preexisting DNA or an incomplete elimination of ^{32}P of intracellular pools of nucleotides.

Figure 3 shows, in addition to the 53S and 18S peaks, a third peak sedimenting at a rate slower than that of 18S. This last peak, also evident in Fig. 1, was identified by hybridization as containing both viral and host DNA's. The absence of this peak from the marker virus, lysed and sedimented in an identical manner, suggests that it is not simply degraded DNA.

In order to estimate accurately the size of the host DNA incorporated into the upper band virus, the virus was lysed in NaOH and centrifuged for 8.5 hours in an alkaline sucrose gradient (14.0 ml) with a Spinco SW40 rotor. The 18S and 16S components of the enzymatically nicked, circular SV40 DNA-II (9) served as markers. The major ^{32}P peak was at 15S, whereas the single linear strand of the viral DNA had a 16S value. In terms of molecular weight, the host strand is 15 percent smaller than the viral strand (10).

To test for contamination of the viral preparations with host DNA, reconstruction experiments were performed in which Vero cells labeled with [^{3}H]thymidine were combined with SV40-infected Vero cells and culture medium. Then SV40 virus was purified as described. There were no detectable peaks of ^{3}H in the virus portion of the second CsCl equilibrium centrifugation.

Only 30 count/min of 10^6 count/min added were present in the lower density virus band. Further, treatment of the virions and pseudovirions with nucleases did not alter the results.

The physical properties of the encapsidated host DNA of the pseudovirions suggest the presence of a linear DNA molecule somewhat smaller than the DNA of the virus. Hybridization has shown that the intact double-stranded circle contains only viral DNA; there was no host DNA present.

The presence of SV40 pseudovirions containing sufficient host nucleic acid for the coding of four to five host proteins suggests an efficient mechanism for gene transfer from one host cell to another.

References and Notes

1. A. M. Kaye and E. Winocour, *J. Mol. Biol.* **24**, 475 (1967); M. R. Michel, B. Hirt, R. Weil, *Proc. Nat. Acad. Sci. U.S.* **58**, 1381 (1967).
2. Abbreviations: SV40 is simian virus 40; SSC is standard saline-citrate, 0.15M NaCl and 0.015M trisodium citrate; 4X SSC is quadruple-strength SSC; TES is *N*-tris(hydroxymethyl)methyl-2-aminoethanesulfonic acid; PM (Denhardt's "preincubation" mixture) contains 0.02 percent bovine serum albumin, 0.02 percent Ficoll, and 0.02 percent polyvinylpyrrolidone; SDS is sodium dodecyl sulfate.
3. Y. Aloni, E. Winocour, L. Sachs, J. Torten, *J. Mol. Biol.* **44**, 333 (1969).
4. R. Radloff, W. Bauer, J. Vinograd, *Proc. Nat. Acad. Sci. U.S.* **57**, 1514 (1967).
5. B. J. McCarthy and B. H. Hoyer, *ibid.* **52**, 915 (1964); K. I. Berns and C. A. Thomas, Jr., *J. Mol. Biol.* **11**, 476 (1965).
6. D. T. Denhardt, *Biochem. Biophys. Res. Commun.* **23**, 641 (1966).
7. M. A. Martin, *J. Virol.* **3**, 119 (1969).
8. K. Yoshiike, *Virology* **34**, 391 (1968).
9. R. Weil and J. Vinograd, *Proc. Nat. Acad. Sci. U.S.* **50**, 730 (1963); J. Vinograd, J. Lebowitz, R. Radloff, R. Watson, P. Laipis, *Proc. Nat. Acad. Sci. U.S.* **53**, 1104 (1965); L. V. Crawford and P. H. Black, *Virology* **24**, 388 (1964).
10. F. W. Studier, *J. Mol. Biol.* **11**, 373 (1965).
11. R. J. Britten, *Carnegie Inst. Wash. Year B.* **67**, 327 (1967–68).
12. We thank Zenia Nimec and Ann Martin for excellent technical assistance.

Morphological Aspects of the Uptake of Simian Virus 40 by Permissive Cells

KLAUS HUMMELER, NATALE TOMASSINI, AND FRANTISEK SOKOL

The morphological aspects of the replication of simian virus 40 (SV40) in permissive cells is well documented (6, 7, 13–15). The preceding events, however, i.e., the mode of uptake by the cells and the intracellular transport of the virus to the nuclear sites of replication, have not been studied. Thus, it is not known whether the SV40 particles lose their protein coat in the cytoplasm while the genome enters the nucleus or whether the particles reach the nucleus morphologically unaltered and the necessary uncoating occurs at nuclear sites of replication.

In the present study, which was designed to investigate the uptake process, highly purified SV40 was used, and susceptible cells were exposed to the virus at a high input multiplicity. The results show that virions penetrate the cellular and nuclear membranes and can be found in the nucleus as early as 1 hr after infection. The mode of uptake and the intracellular pathways of SV40 are also described.

MATERIALS AND METHODS

Cells. Primary African green monkey kidney cells (AGMK) were cultured in 30-ml plastic flasks at 37 C. CV-1 cells, a continuous cell line isolated from AGMK cells (9), were grown in 1-liter Blake bottles in an atmosphere of 4% CO_2. The growth and maintenance media used for both cell types were described previously (5).

Virus. The LP 4 large-plaque variant of the RH 911 strain of SV40 was used in all experiments. The preparation of virus pools in monolayer cultures of CV-1 cells and the assay of the virus by the plaque technique were described previously (4, 5). Virus pools used in the present study contained an average of 2×10^8 plaque-forming units (PFU) per ml.

Purification and concentration of virus. SV40 was concentrated and purified by a procedure outlined before (5), except that treatment with trypsin was omitted because it was found to decrease the infectivity of the preparation. To separate fully infectious SV40 from noninfectious, incomplete viral forms (16–18) and from coreless viral shells (2), the purified virus was centrifuged to equilibrium in CsCl solution with an average density of 1.30 g/cc in the SW 50 rotor of a Spinco centrifuge at 5 C and 130,000 × g for 24 hr. The band of fully infectious virus located at a density of 1.34 g/cc was collected and freed from CsCl by dialysis against 0.13 M NaCl-0.05 M tris-(hydroxymethyl)aminomethane (Tris) at pH 7.8 (NT buffer). The infectivity of the purified virus was stabilized by the addition of 5% fetal calf serum, and all preparations were used within 24 hr for infection of AGMK cells. The infectivity titers of these preparations ranged from 9×10^{10} to 19×10^{10} PFU/ml. The purified virus had a 260/280 nm optical density ratio of 1.37 to 1.39, indicating the absence of coreless virus shells (10). It was previously determined that 1 mg of purified SV40 corresponds to 3.85 OD_{260} units (10) and that the molecular weight of the virus is 17.3×10^6 daltons (1). By using these data, it was calculated that the purified virus preparations used in the present study contained 10 to 20 virions per PFU.

Infection of cell cultures and electron microscopy. Cultures of AGMK cells were infected at a multiplicity of about 1,000. At the intervals indicated below, the inoculum was decanted and the cultures were washed three times with phosphate-buffered saline (PBS). Subsequently, the infected monolayers were fixed in situ, dehydrated, and embedded as described previously (8). The infection of the cultures was interrupted at 10, 30, and 45 min, and at 1 and 2 hr. After removal of inoculum and washing, medium was added to some cultures which were harvested at 4, 6, 24, and 48 hr.

Thin sections were doubly stained with uranyl acetate and lead citrate and were viewed in an electron-microscope at a magnification of 10,500.

RESULTS

For the purpose of illustrating the results of this investigation, the 10-min, 2-hr, and 24-hr intervals were selected because they demonstrated the pertinent features. At 10 min after infection, virus particles were found attached to the plasmalemma and inside the cytoplasm. In Fig. 1 the attachment of the virus particles on the cell membrane can be seen. They are aligned along the plasmalemma; aggregates were rarely observed. Actual uptake of the virus by the cell occurred by two mechanisms: (i) engulfment of single virus particles and (ii) formation of pinocytotic vesicles containing several of them. The

first mechanism, or monopinocytosis, can be seen in Fig. 2 and 3. After engulfment, the cell membrane seemed to close tightly behind the particle, and the newly acquired membrane increased the diameter of the virus by 15 nm. Such a particle is demonstrated in Fig. 4. It should be pointed out that the efficacy of uptake was low. Numerous particles were consistently found still attached to the plasma membrane many hours after exposure.

The second mechanism of uptake is demonstrated in Fig. 4 and 5. In the particular cell system under investigation, it was rarely seen. Several virus particles were engulfed by the cell membrane, forming pinocytotic vesicles. The beginning of the process can be seen in Fig. 4 and the end result in Fig. 5. Whether particles can escape from these vesicles into the cytoplasm by

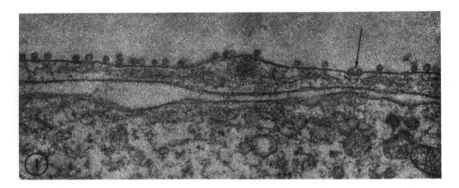

Fig. 1. *SV40 particles attached to the plasma membrane at 10 min after infection. Beginning pinocytosis is marked by the arrow.* × *73,500.*

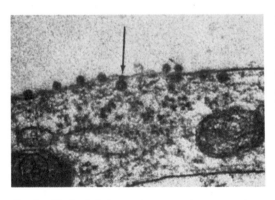 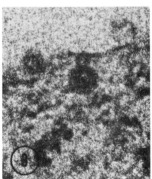

Fig. 2 and 3. *Single SV40 particle near completion of pinocytosis at 10 min after infection. The cell membrane envelops the particle tightly and is in the process of closing behind it. Fig. 2,* × *73,500. Fig. 3,* × *210,000.*

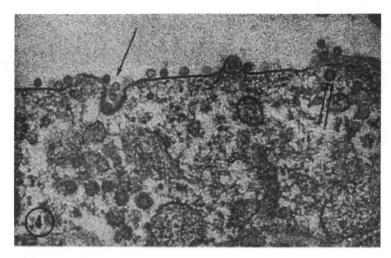

Fig. 4. *Modes of SV40 uptake at 10 min after infection. Pinocytosis of several particles on the left (single arrow), and completed uptake of single particle on the right (double arrow). The diameter of this particle has increased from 40 to 55 nm.* × *73,500.*

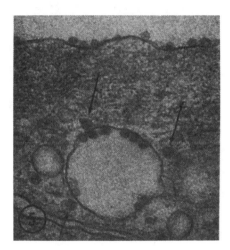

Fig. 5. *Pinocytotic vesicle containing several SV40 particles at 10 min after infection. Release of single particles from vesicle into the cytoplasm was not observed, but particles larger in diameter can be seen close to the vesicle membrane (arrows).* × *73,500.*

the monopinocytotic mechanism responsible for the uptake could not be observed directly, but several particles with increased diameters were evident in the cytoplasm near the membrane of the vesicle in Fig. 5. Enveloped single virus particles were found occasionally in the proximity of the nucleus at 10 min after infection.

Virus particles devoid of the membrane acquired at the initial uptake were found in the nucleus at 1 hr after infection, although they were seen most frequently at the 2-hr interval. The actual mechanism of passage through the nuclear membranes was difficult to determine. It seems, however, that the acquired membrane fused with the outer nuclear membrane, as can be seen in Fig. 6 and 7, and that only the original virus particle proceeded into the nucleus to cause morphological alterations of the nuclear membranes. All particles found in the nucleus had the same diameter as the original infecting virus, namely, 40 nm. In Fig. 8, two virus particles in the nucleus seemed to have passed the nuclear membrane barrier recently. In both cases, the nuclear membranes are disturbed in proximity to the particles. Occasionally, groups of virus particles were found in the nucleus (Fig. 9 and 10). The process of uncoating seems to start very early; at least, some morphological evidence of that phenomenon can be seen in Fig. 9 and 10. Morphologically discernible virus particles could not be found in the nucleus at 4 hr after infection.

Morphological evidence of viral replication became evident at 24 hr after infection, as is demonstrated in Fig. 11. All further events of virus development proceeded as described previously (14).

149

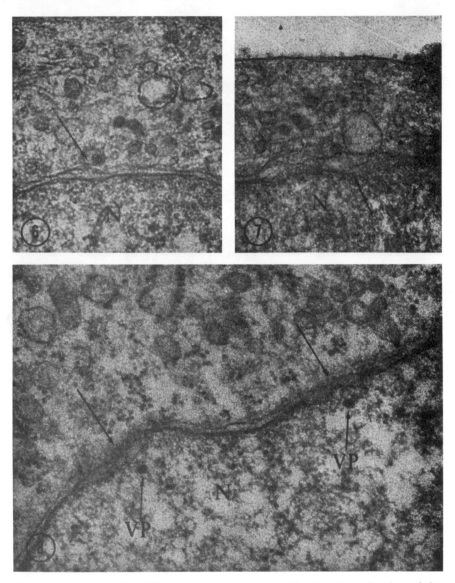

FIG. 6. *Interaction of engulfed SV40 with outer nuclear membrane at 2 hr after infection. Particle attached to or fused with outer nuclear membrane (arrow), losing its cell membrane in the process. Structure of outer nuclear membrane becomes disturbed. N, nucleus.* × 73,500.

FIG. 7. *Same as in Fig. 6. Both nuclear membranes show alteration of their fine structure.*

FIG. 8. *Two SV40 particles in the nucleus after penetration of the nuclear membrane, 2 hr after infection. Morphology of the nuclear membranes is altered at point of penetration (arrows), and the particles have regained their original diameter, 40 nm, indicating loss of cell membranes during process of penetration. N, nucleus; VP, virus particles.* × 73,500.

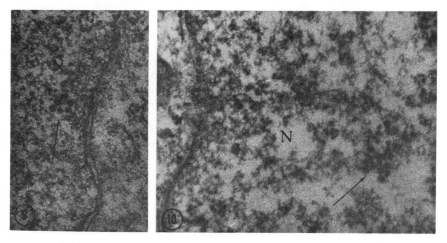

FIG. 9 and 10. *Groups of SV40 particles in the nucleus at 2 hr after infection. Some particles appear less elec tron-dense than others, possibly indicating the beginning of the uncoating process.*

DISCUSSION

To facilitate morphological studies on the process of infection of permissive cells by SV40, highly purified virus, from which the bulk of noninfectious, incomplete particles had been eliminated, was used at a high multiplicity of input. Under those circumstances, virus attachment to the plasma membrane seemed to occur almost immediately, all input virus showing a remarkable affinity for the cell membrane. Only a relatively small fraction of the attached particles entered the cell. The remaining virus stayed attached to the plasma membrane and could be observed in this position hours after the initial contact, the time when most of them seemed to undergo a process of degeneration.

The most prevalent mode of entry was a pinocytosis of single particles, or monopinocytosis. After this had been accomplished, the virus particles were easily recognized in the cytoplasm by the addition of the extra membrane adhering closely to the particle itself. This process resulted in an increase of diameter from 40 to 55 nm. Pinocytoses of several particles into larger vesicles were seen rarely in the system under investigation. The uptake of single virus particles from these vesicles into the cytoplasm, however, cannot be excluded, and indirect evidence pointed to its occurrence. Thus, such particles may also contribute to the infectious process. Particles without the additional membrane were never found in the cytoplasm, and, therefore, direct transfer of SV40 through the plasmalemma with-

out engulfment seemed not to be a likely mechanism of infection.

The engulfed particles passed into the nucleus by fusion of their cell-acquired coat with the nuclear membranes and subsequent injection into the nucleus with loss of the acquired cell membrane in the process. These mechanisms were similar to those found by Mattern et al. (12) with polyoma virus, except that polyoma virus was found only in the nuclear membrane interspace. The failure to observe polyoma virus in the nucleus may have been a result of the relatively low input multiplicity used, because the efficiency of transfer of SV40 from the cytoplasm to the nucleus was low even at high multiplicities of infection.

Invasion of the nucleus was seen as early as 1 hr after infection. Preliminary radioautographic experiments with ³H-thymidine-labeled SV40 also indicated the presence of viral deoxyribonucleic acid (DNA) in the nucleus at this time (*unpublished observations*). The greatest number of intranuclear SV40 was found at 2 hr after infection, and morphological evidence indicated that uncoating of the virus began almost immediately upon arrival at the nuclear uncoating site. This is further supported by the fact that at 4 hr after infection intranuclear invading virus was no longer found. Biochemical studies on the uptake of SV40 by permissive cells and the intracellular uncoating were in agreement with these morphological findings (2).

The efficiency with which parental virus is

151

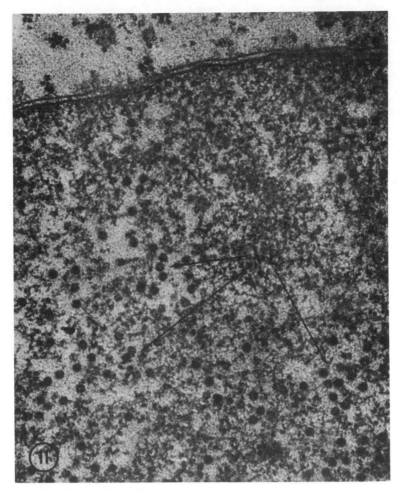

Fig. 11. *Nucleus of cell infected with SV40 24 hr previously. Viral progeny is apparent. N, nucleus; VP, virus particles.* × 73,500.

seemingly uncoated in the nucleus raises the question why the progeny virus is impervious to this process. This may be due to an inhibition of the synthesis, or activity, of nuclear uncoating enzymes after the start of viral DNA replication, or the progeny virus may have a protein coat sufficiently different from the infecting particles to protect it against uncoating enzymes. The observations by Levinthal et al. (11) and Oshiro et al. (15) that virus-specific ferritin-labeled antibody did not tag intranuclear virus but was readily bound to intracytoplasmic virus particles would speak for a different coat antigen on nuclear progeny virus, which is either lost or changed upon leaving the nucleus. Thus, the different antigenic surface or configuration of the viral coat may protect progeny virus against uncoating enzymes in the nucleus.

ACKNOWLEDGMENTS

This investigation was supported by Public Health Service research grants AI-04911 from the National Institute of Allergy and Infectious Diseases and CA-10594 from the National Cancer Institute.

The technical assistance of Mary K. Sheehan is gratefully acknowledged.

LITERATURE CITED

1. Anderer, F. A., H. D. Schlumberger, M. A. Koch, H. Frank, and H. T. Eggers. 1967. Structure of simian virus 40. II. Symmetry and components of the virus particle. Virology 32:511–523.
2. Barbanti-Brodano, G., P. Swetly, and H. Koprowski. 1970. Early events in the infection of permissive cells with simian virus 40: adsorption, penetration, and uncoating. J. Virol. 6:78–86.
3. Black, P. H., E. M. Crawford, and L. V. Crawford. 1964. The purification of simian virus 40. Virology 24:381–387.
4. Carp, R. I., and R. V. Gilden. 1966. A comparison of the replication cycles of simian virus 40 in human diploid and African green monkey kidney cells. Virology 28:150–162.
5. Carp, R. I., G. Sauer, and F. Sokol. 1969. The effect of actinomycin D on the transcription and replication of simian virus 40 deoxyribonucleic acid. Virology 37:214–226.
6. Gaylord, W. H., Jr., and G. D. Hsiung. 1961. The vacuolating virus of monkeys. II. Virus morphology and intranuclear distribution with some histochemical observations. J. Exp. Med. 114:987–996.
7. Granboulan, N., P. Tournier, R. Wicker, and W. Bernhard 1963. An electron microscope study of the development of SV40 virus. J. Cell Biol. 17:423–441.
8. Hummeler, K., N. Tomassini, and D. Zajac. 1969. Early events in herpes simplex virus infection: a radioautographic study. J. Virol. 4:67–74.
9. Jensen, F. C., A. J. Girardi, R. V. Gilden, and H. Koprowski.

10. Koch, M. A., H. J. Eggers, F. A. Anderer, H. D. Schlumberger, and H. Frank. 1967. Structure of simian virus 40. I. Purification and physical characterization of the virus particle. Virology 32:503–510.
11. Levinthal, J. D., R. Wicker, and J. C. Cerottini. 1967. Study of intracellular SV40 antigen by indirect immunoferritin technique. Virology 31:555–558.
12. Mattern, C. F. T., K. K. Takemoto, and W. A. Wendell. 1966. Replication of polyoma virus in mouse embryo cells: Electronmicroscopic observations. Virology 30:242–256.
13. Mayor, H. D., R. M. Jamison, L. E. Jordan, and S. McGregor. 1966. The influence of p-fluorophenylalanine, puromycin and actinomycin on the development of simian papovavirus (SV40). Exp. Mol. Pathol. 5:245–262.
14. Mayor, H. D., S. E. Stinebaugh, R. M. Jamison, L. E. Jordan, and J. L. Melnick. 1962. Immunofluorescent, cytochemical and microcytological studies on the growth of the simian vacuolating virus (SV40) in tissue culture. Exp. Mol. Pathol. 1:397–416.
15. Oshiro, L. S., H. M. Rose, C. Morgan, and K. C. Hsu. 1967. Electron microscopic study of the development of simian virus 40 by use of ferritin-labeled antibodies. J. Virol. 1:384–399.
16. Uchida, S., K. Yoshiika, S. Watanabe, and A. Furuno. 1968. Antigen-forming defective viruses of simian virus 40. Virology 34:1–8.
17. Yoshiike, K. 1968. Studies on DNA from low-density particles of SV40. I. Heterogeneous defective virions produced by successive undiluted passages. Virology 34:391–401.
18. Yoshiike, K. 1968. Studies on DNA from low density particles of SV40. II. Noninfectious virions associated with a large-plaque variant. Virology 34:402–409.

Early Events in the Infection of Permissive Cells with Simian Virus 40: Adsorption, Penetration, and Uncoating

GIUSEPPE BARBANTI-BRODANO, PETER SWETLY, AND HILARY KOPROWSKI

In a previous report (18), we showed the resistance to superinfection with simian virus 40 (SV-40) and SV40 deoxyribonucleic acid (DNA) of SV40-transformed nonpermissive cells. In addition, we found that SV40-transformed permissive cells are resistant to superinfection with SV40, but susceptible to SV40 DNA. Hence, the infection of SV40-transformed permissive cells with intact virus is probably blocked at an early stage, before the replication of viral DNA occurs.

A comparison of the early events of infection in SV40-transformed permissive cells with the same phase of the infectious cycle in nontransformed permissive cells may elucidate the nature of this block.

The early events of cell-virus interaction in nontransformed permissive cells have not been extensively investigated. The present report describes the adsorption, penetration, and uncoating of SV40 in such cells.

MATERIALS AND METHODS

Cells. Primary and secondary African green monkey kidney (AGMK) cells and CV-1 cells, a continuous line derived from AGMK cells (8), were grown in Eagle's basal medium supplemented with 10% fetal bovine serum (FBS). They were maintained, after infection with SV40, in the same medium supplemented with 2% FBS.

Virus. The Rh 911 strain of SV40 was grown in CV-1 cells as described previously (18).

Labeling of the virus. Monolayer cultures of CV-1 cells were infected at an input multiplicity of 50 plaque-forming units (PFU) per cell. To prepare virus isotopically labeled in the DNA, the medium was removed 15 hr after infection and replaced with fresh medium containing 5 μc of ³H-thymidine (specific activity, 17 c/mmole; New England Nuclear Corp., Boston, Mass.) per ml. To prepare virus isotopically labeled in the proteins, the medium was removed 30 hr after infection and replaced with fresh medium containing one-third of the normal amount of cold leucine (17 μg/ml) and 5 μc of ³H-leucine (specific activity, 40 c/mmole; Schwarz BioResearch Inc., Orangeburg, N.Y.) per ml. The infected cultures were harvested 72 to 96 hr after infection, when the cytopathic effect involved 75 to 100% of the cells. The virus was purified as described previously (18), except that treatment with trypsin was omitted because it was found to decrease the infectivity.

When the purified virus preparations were stained with potassium phosphotungstate and examined with an electron microscope, they were seen to contain 3 to 5% coreless virions. After equilibrium centrifugation in a CsCl solution (106,000 × g for 20 hr), 93% of the radioactivity contained in the purified virus preparations was recovered in a single band located at a density range of 1.30 to 1.38 g/cc. The density at the peak of the band was 1.34 g/cc. The ³H-thymidine-labeled and purified virus contained 2.5 × 10⁶ counts per min per ml and 6.5 × 10¹⁰ PFU per ml. The ³H-leucine-labeled virus contained 1.6 × 10⁶ counts per min per ml and 3.4 × 10¹⁰ PFU per ml.

Isolation of ³H-thymidine-labeled SV40 DNA. SV40 DNA was extracted from a ³H-thymidine-labeled and purified virus preparation as described previously (18).

Infection of cells with labeled and purified virus. Confluent monolayer cultures of AGMK cells were infected with ³H-thymidine- or ³H-leucine-labeled SV40. The virus was adsorbed for 2 hr at 37 C. The inoculum was removed and the cell monolayer was washed three times with phosphate-buffered saline (PBS). After the addition of maintenance medium, the cells were incubated at 37 C. (The term "after infection" used in the description of all experiments refers *not* to the time interval after the 2-hr adsorption but to the time interval after the addition of virus.)

Disruption of cells and fractionation of cellular components. Three techniques were used for the disruption of cells and the fractionation of cellular components.

Method A. At various intervals after infection, cell monolayers were washed three times with PBS. The cells were dispersed with trypsin and sedimented by centrifugation at $1,000 \times g$ for 4 min. The pelleted cells were suspended in PBS, sedimented again, resuspended in 1 ml of a 0.25 M sucrose solution, and homogenized in a glass tissue grinder (Ten-Broeck type; Bellco Glass, Inc., Vineland, N.J.) at 0 C until more than 90% of the cells were broken. The cell homogenate was fractionated by differential centrifugation at 4 C into three fractions: a nuclear fraction (sediment obtained after centrifugation at $600 \times g$ for 5 min), a large-granule fraction containing mitochondria and lysosomes (sediment obtained after centrifugation of the $600 \times g$ supernatant fluid at $10,000 \times g$ for 30 min), and a cytoplasmic supernatant (supernatant fluid obtained after centrifugation at $10,000 \times g$ for 30 min). This procedure was similar to that described by Silverstein and Dales (17).

Method B. Cells were harvested as described in method A and sedimented at $1,000 \times g$ for 4 min at 4 C. The pelleted cells were washed once with NTM buffer [0.14 M NaCl, 0.01 M tris(hydroxymethyl)-aminomethane (Tris)-chloride, 0.0015 M $MgCl_2$, pH 7.4] and sedimented again. The cells were disrupted by resuspending them in 2 ml of 0.5% Nonidet P-40 (NP-40) nonionic detergent (Shell Chemical Co.) in NTM buffer (1, 13). After incubation at 0 C for 10 min with occasional shaking, the suspension was centrifuged at $1,600 \times g$ for 2 min at 4 C. The cytoplasmic supernatant fluid was decanted, and the sedimented nuclei were washed once in PBS. Nuclei from 65 to 80% of the cells contained in the original cell cultures were recovered by this method. No contamination with cytoplasmic components could be detected when the final nuclear preparation was examined by phase-contrast microscopy.

Method C. Nuclei were isolated according to a procedure described by Penman (15).

Isopycnic centrifugation in CsCl solution of SV40 recovered from nuclei of infected cells. Nuclei isolated from infected AGMK cells were suspended in 0.9 ml of 0.5% NP-40 in NTM buffer. A 0.1-ml amount of 10% sodium deoxycholate (DOC) in distilled water was added, and the mixture was incubated for 10 min at 37 C. The lysed nuclei were mixed with 4 ml of 45.5% (w/v) CsCl solution in 0.02 M Tris-chloride, pH 7.4 (average density, 1.33 g/cc), and centrifuged for 20 hr at 4 C at $106,000 \times g$ in the SW 39 rotor of a Spinco centrifuge. Three-drop fractions were then collected from the bottom of the tubes and assayed for radioactivity. The density of the fractions was calculated from the refractive index (7), determined in an Abbé refractometer.

Rate zonal centrifugation in alkaline sucrose gradients. Nuclei isolated from infected AGMK cells were suspended in 0.3 ml of 0.5% DOC in distilled water and layered on top of 5 to 20% (w/v) linear sucrose density gradients (5 ml) in 0.8 M NaCl and 0.2 M NaOH (pH 12.4). The contents of the tubes were centrifuged at $106,000 \times g$ for 90 min at 4 C in the SW 39 rotor of a Spinco centrifuge. Three-drop fractions were collected from the bottom of the tubes and the radioactivity was assayed.

Treatment with deoxyribonuclease and phosphodiesterase. Cytoplasmic and nuclear fractions of AGMK cells infected with ^{3}H-thymidine-labeled SV40 were treated with 200 μg of pancreatic deoxyribonuclease per ml (deoxyribonuclease I, Sigma Chemical Co., St. Louis, Mo.) and 0.1 unit of phosphodiesterase per ml (Sigma Chemical Co.) in the presence of 0.02 M $MgSO_4$ for 30 min at 37 C. The nuclease-resistant material was then precipitated with trichloroacetic acid, and the radioactivity was determined. The uncoating of viral DNA was evaluated according to Joklik (9) on the basis of the amount of nuclease-sensitive acid-precipitable radioactivity present in the cells after infection with ^{3}H-thymidine-labeled SV40.

The presence of NP-40 and DOC in the cellular fractions did not inhibit the action of nucleases, as has also been reported for adenovirus type 5 (10), and did not affect the buoyant density of the viral particles.

Determination of radioactivity. Total radioactivity was determined by addition of 20- or 40-μliter samples to glass-fiber filters (934 AH; diameter, 2.4 cm; H. Reeve Angel & Co., Inc., Clifton, N.J.). The filters were dried, and the radioactivity was counted in 10 ml of Liquifluor (New England Nuclear Corp.) diluted in toluene. The radioactivity of the acid-precipitable material was determined by the addition of 30 μg of carrier yeast ribonucleic acid per ml and trichloroacetic acid to a concentration of 5%. The samples were kept at 0 C for 1 hr. The precipitate was collected by filtration through glass-fiber filters and dried. The radioactivity was measured by counting for 10 min in a Packard liquid scintillation spectrometer.

RESULTS

Kinetics of adsorption of SV40 onto AGMK cells. Within 15 min, 30% of the input radioactivity of the ^{3}H-thymidine-labeled virus became cell associated. The rate of adsorption then reached a plateau, 50% of the total input radioactivity being adsorbed 2 hr after infection (Fig. 1).

To determine whether SV40 was bound firmly to the receptors of the cell membrane, AGMK cells infected with ^{3}H-thymidine-labeled virus were harvested 10 min after infection and disrupted; the cell homogenate was then centrifuged in a neutral CsCl density gradient (Fig. 2). The bulk of the cell-associated radioactivity banded at the density of 1.27 g/cc, indicating binding of the virus to lipoprotein-containing cell components, and only 10% of the radioactivity was recovered

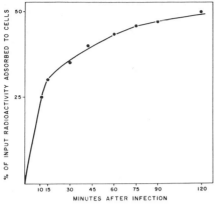

FIG. 1. *Kinetics of adsorption of SV40 onto AGMK cells. Confluent monolayers containing 3 × 10⁶ AGMK cells were infected with ³H-thymidine-labeled SV40 at an input multiplicity of 100 PFU/cell (input radioactivity, 1.5 × 10⁴ counts per min per culture). The infected cultures were incubated at 37 C. At intervals after infection, the inoculum was removed; the cells were washed three times with PBS and harvested into a final volume of 2 ml. The acid-precipitable radioactivity contained in the cell suspension was then determined.*

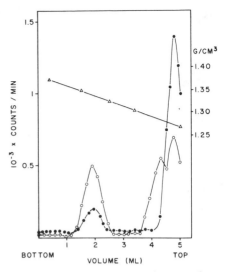

FIG. 2. *Association of SV40 with cell membrane components. Confluent monolayers containing 6 × 10⁶ AGMK cells were infected with ³H-thymidine-labeled SV40 at an input multiplicity of 100 PFU/cell (input radioactivity, 3 × 10⁴ counts per min per culture). At 10 min after infection, the cells were washed three times with PBS and scraped into 5 ml of PBS. The cell suspension was then centrifuged at 1,000 × g for 5 min at 4 C. The sedimented cells were resuspended in 1 ml of RSB buffer of Penman (15) and broken with 25 strokes in a tight-fitting Dounce homogenizer. One-half of the cell homogenate was layered on top of a pre-formed linear CsCl density gradient (average density, 1.33 g/cc) and centrifuged at 106,000 × g for 5 hr at 4 C in the SW 39 rotor of a Spinco L centrifuge. The other half of the cell homogenate was incubated with 0.5% DOC at 37 C for 20 min before layering on top of the gradient. Fractions of 3 drops were collected from the bottom of the gradients, and the radioactivity was determined. Symbols: △, density at 25 C; ●, radioactivity of ³H-thymidine; ○, radioactivity of ³H-thymidine after treatment with DOC.*

in the form of free virus banding at a density of 1.34 g/cc. After treatment of the cell homogenate with DOC, 33% of the radioactivity recovered before treatment at a density of 1.27 g/cc was shifted to the density of free SV40 particles.

Distribution of SV40 and its components in infected cells. The distribution of SV40 in the infected cells was determined in the following way. Cells infected with ³H-thymidine- or ³H-leucine-labeled virus were harvested at intervals after infection, disrupted, and fractionated. The radioactivity contained in the acid-precipitable cellular fractions was then determined. The results shown in Table 1 indicate that at 30 min after infection most of the cytoplasmic radioactivity was associated with large granules, although an appreciable quantity of label was also found at that time in the nuclei. The relative amount of ³H-leucine radioactivity recovered from the nuclei was higher than that of ³H-thymidine. This observation was confirmed in repeated experiments.

At 60 min after infection, the radioactivity associated with the nuclei increased significantly, whereas that associated with the large-granule fraction decreased correspondingly. The transfer of cytoplasmic radioactivity from the large-granule fraction to the nuclei continued for up to

120 min after infection. Less than 10% of the total intracellular radioactivity was recovered in the cytoplasmic supernatant fluid between 30 and 120 min after infection.

Kinetics of uncoating of SV40 in the cytoplasm and nuclei of infected cells. The distribution of the ³H-leucine- and ³H-thymidine-labeled viral components between the cytoplasm and the nuclei of infected cells was determined for the period from 0.5 to 24 hr after infection. At the same time, so that the uncoating of SV40 in the cytoplasm and in the nuclei might be investigated, the sensitivity

TABLE 1. *Distribution of SV40 in different fractions of infected cells*[a]

Fraction	Percentage of cell-associated radioactivity at various intervals after infection					
	^{3}H-thymidine			^{3}H-leucine		
	30 min	60 min	120 min	30 min	60 min	120 min
Nuclei...........	10	32	50	36	58	66
Large granules...	84	64	43	59	36	26
10,000 × *g* supernatant fluid...	6	4	7	5	6	6

[a] Monolayer cultures containing 6×10^6 AGMK cells were infected with ^{3}H-thymidine- or ^{3}H-leucine-labeled SV40 at an input multiplicity of 2 PFU/cell (input radioactivity, 6×10^2 counts per min per culture). Cells were harvested at intervals after infection, homogenized, and fractionated by method A described in Materials and Methods. The acid-precipitable radioactivity contained in the fractions was then determined.

of the viral DNA to the degrading action of nucleases was determined (Fig. 3).

The time dependence of the distribution of the ^{3}H-leucine and ^{3}H-thymidine viral radioactivity in the nuclei and in the cytoplasm followed a similar pattern. At 2.5 hr after infection, approximately 60% of both the ^{3}H-thymidine and ^{3}H-leucine cell-associated radioactivity was found in the nuclei. Between 2.5 and 4 hr after infection, the release of both radioactive precursors from the nuclei was accompanied by a complementary increase in the radioactivity recovered in the cytoplasmic fraction. Later, a gradual decrease in acid-precipitable radioactivity of both the nuclear and cytoplasmic fractions was observed. Between 3 and 5% of the cell-associated ^{3}H-thymidine or ^{3}H-leucine acid-precipitable radioactivities were recovered in the medium at any time between 2 and 24 hr after infection. About one-third of the acid-precipitable ^{3}H-thymidine radioactivity contained in the medium was degraded by the action of nucleases.

SV40 DNA contained in the cytoplasmic fraction (Fig. 3a) displayed sensitivity to nucleases as early as 0.5 hr after infection. This sensitivity reached a maximum at 4 hr, when 50% of the acid-precipitable ^{3}H-thymidine radioactivity contained in the cytoplasm was digested by nucleases. In contrast, the intranuclear viral DNA was almost completely refractory to the action of nucleases up to 1.5 hr after infection (Fig. 3b), whereas at 2.5 hr and later about 60% of the acid-precipitable ^{3}H-thymidine radioactivity became sensitive to the action of the enzymes.

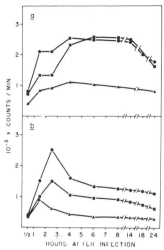

FIG. 3. *Distribution of SV40 proteins and SV40 DNA between the cytoplasm and the nuclei of infected cells and sensitivity of the viral DNA to nucleases. Monolayer cultures containing 6×10^6 AGMK cells were infected with ^{3}H-thymidine- or ^{3}H-leucine-labeled SV40 at an input multiplicity of 100 PFU/cell (input radioactivity, 3×10^4 counts per min per culture). Cells were harvested at intervals after infection, and the nuclei were separated from the cytoplasm by method B, described in Materials and Methods. The acid-precipitable radioactivity contained in the cytoplasmic (a) and in the nuclear (b) fractions was determined. In cells infected with ^{3}H-thymidine-labeled virus, the acid-precipitable radioactivity of the fractions was determined also after treatment with deoxyribonuclease and phosphodiesterase. Each point represents mean values from five independent experiments. Symbols:* ●, *[3]H-leucine radioactivity;* ■, *[3]H-thymidine radioactivity;* ▲, *[3]H-thymidine radioactivity refractory to the action of deoxyribonuclease and phosphodiesterase.*

Isolation of SV40 particles from nuclei of infected cells. The experiments described above have shown that both viral proteins and viral DNA can be recovered from the nuclei of infected cells soon after infection. To determine whether intact virions penetrate the nuclei, AGMK cells were infected with ^{3}H-thymidine- or ^{3}H-leucine-labeled SV40 and were harvested at intervals after infection; their nuclei were then analyzed for the presence of SV40 particles (Fig. 4 and 5). Between 0.5 and 2.5 hr after infection, both ^{3}H-thymidine and ^{3}H-leucine radioactivity recovered from the disrupted nuclei banded after equilibrium density gradient centrifugation at a density of 1.34 g/cc. Later, the density of the ^{3}H-thymidine-labeled viral components recovered

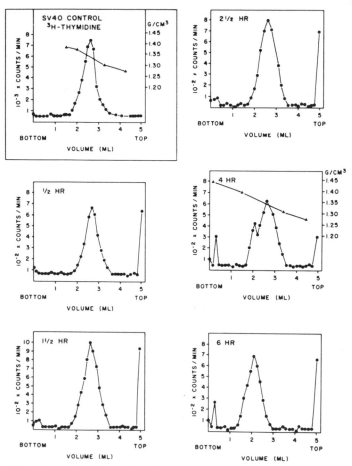

FIG. 4. *Isolation of parental SV40 from nuclei of infected cells. Confluent monolayer cultures containing 6 × 10⁶ AGMK cells were infected with ³H-thymidine-labeled SV40 at an input multiplicity of 100 PFU/cell (input radioactivity, 3 × 10⁴ counts per min per culture). At intervals after infection cells were harvested, and the nuclei were isolated by method B, described in Materials and Methods. Nuclei were disrupted and analyzed by equilibrium centrifugation in CsCl density gradients. In parallel, purified and labeled SV40 preparations used for the infection of cells were analyzed. Symbols:* ▲, *density at 25 C;* ●, *total radioactivity.*

from the nuclei shifted gradually to a density of 1.37 g/cc. A minor component banding at a density of 1.43 g/cc could also be detected at 4 hr after infection (Fig. 4). Between 4 and 6 hr after infection, the density of the ³H-leucine-labeled material recovered from the nuclei shifted gradually from 1.34 to 1.30 g/cc (Fig. 5). About 20% of both the ³H-thymidine and ³H-leucine radioactivity contained in the nuclei was found at the top of the gradients.

The results of these experiments indicate that from 0.5 to 2.5 hr after infection intact virions can be recovered from the nuclei of infected AGMK cells. Between 2.5 and 4 hr after infection, intranuclear virions started to be uncoated. The protein coat of the virus was completely removed from the viral genome, and the parental DNA became associated with either cellular or newly synthesized viral proteins.

Fate of parental SV40 DNA in the nuclei of

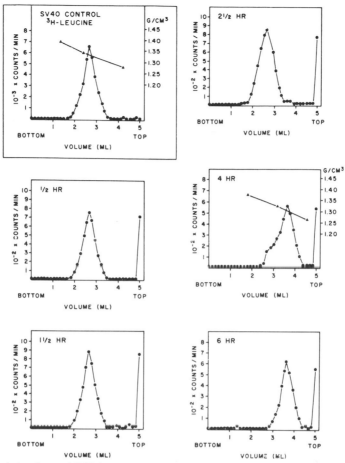

FIG. 5. *Isolation of parental SV40 from nuclei of infected cells. Confluent monolayer cultures containing 6 × 10⁶ AGMK cells were infected with ³H-leucine-labeled SV40 at an input multiplicity of 100 PFU/cell (input radioactivity, 3 × 10⁴ counts per min per culture). Experimental conditions and symbols are as described in the legend to Fig. 4.*

infected cells. The state of intranuclear SV40 DNA was investigated by rate zonal centrifugation in alkaline sucrose gradients of nuclei isolated from cells harvested at various intervals after infection.

The sedimentation properties of the intranuclear viral DNA were compared with those of ³H-thymidine-labeled SV40 DNA extracted from purified virus preparations (Fig. 6). After denaturation in alkaline solution, component I of SV40 DNA (2) has a sedimentation coefficient of 53S [the same as that described for the DNA of the related polyoma virus (19)], whereas com-

ponent II of SV40 DNA (2) is usually separated in two single-stranded DNA fractions sedimenting at 18S and 16S (19). However, under the conditions of centrifugation used in these experiments, the single-stranded circular and linear forms of component II were not resolved.

Viral DNA extracted from the purified virions contained about 90% of component I and 10% of component II, whereas intranuclear viral DNA isolated from the cells as early as 2.5 hr after infection contained 34% of component I, 26% of component II, and 25% of an unidentified com-

159

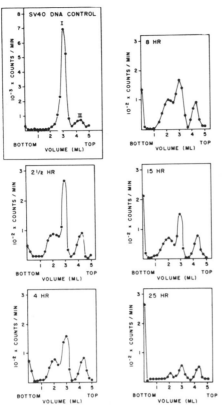

FIG. 6. *Fate of parental SV40 DNA in the nuclei of infected cells. Monolayer cultures containing 6 × 10⁶ AGMK cells were infected with ³H-thymidine-labeled SV40 at an input multiplicity of 50 PFU/cell (input radioactvity, 1.5 × 10⁴ counts per min per culture). Nuclei were isolated from cells at intervals after infection by method B, described in Materials and Methods. The nuclear suspension was layered on top of an alkaline sucrose density gradient, centrifuged, and analyzed as described in Materials and Methods. Sedimentation coefficients were determined as described by Martin and Ames (12).*

ponent sedimenting at 76*S*. The band corresponding to the 76*S* component was always broader than those corresponding to component I and component II, indicating a high degree of heterogeneity of the 76*S* component. Up to 15 hr after infection, the relative proportion of component II and of the 76*S* component, as well as of the DNA sedimenting to the bottom of the gradient, increased while that of component I

decreased. At 25 hr after infection, a decrease in the total amount of component I, component II, and the 76*S* component was observed, and the amount of DNA sedimenting to the bottom of the gradient was markedly increased.

DISCUSSION

As previously reported for different SV40 mutants (14), the adsorption of SV40 to permissive cells is a rapid process, and 50% of the input virus is adsorbed within 2 hr after infection. The association of viral radioactivity at 10 min after infection with lipoprotein-containing cell components suggests that the virus adsorption is mediated by a combination of the viral particles with cellular receptors. The binding of the virus to the cell membrane is strong, because the virus-receptor complex is not dissociated in a CsCl solution and viral particles are only partially released after treatment with DOC. It is possible, however, that intracellular components are also bound to the virus as early as 10 min after infection, because intracytoplasmic virions can be detected in this phase of infection by electron microscopic techniques (6).

The association of most of the intracellular virus with the large cytoplasmic granules soon after infection indicates that, after penetration, viral particles are not in a free state in the cytoplasm of the infected cells, but are bound to discrete cytoplasmic structures, probably pinocytotic vacuoles formed after the engulfment of the virions into the cells. Similar electron microscopic observations have been described for most of the animal viruses (3), as well as for SV40 (6).

The simultaneous shift of viral proteins and viral DNA from the cytoplasm to the nuclei, observed between 0.5 and 2.5 hr after infection, indicates that the whole virus penetrates the nucleus. Intact virions were indeed recovered from the nuclei. The possibility of cytoplasmic contamination of the nuclear fraction, and of virus particles being attached to the nuclear membranes rather than penetrating the nucleus, was excluded by the use of the Penman method for isolation of the nuclei. When this procedure, which strips away the "contaminating" cytoplasm and the outer membrane from the nucleus (5), was followed, the amount of SV40 virions recovered from the nuclei was similar to that obtained by other methods. These findings were confirmed by electron microscopic observations of intact virus particles present in the nucleoplasm of AGMK cells as early as 1 hr after infection with SV40 (6).

The sensitivity of the intranuclear viral DNA to nucleases indicates that the uncoating of the virus is carried out within the nucleus. In fact, the intranuclear uncoating seems to be an endogenous process starting from intact viral particles, since the virions in the nuclei of infected AGMK cells show the same size and morphology (6) and have the same buoyant density in CsCl as those contained in purified SV40 preparations.

At present, it is difficult to decide whether cytoplasm plays any role in the uncoating of SV40. As we have observed, the cytoplasmic viral DNA is sensitive to nucleases as early as 0.5 hr after infection. The viral coat proteins released are rapidly transferred to the nucleus, as indicated by the high ^{3}H-leucine to ^{3}H-thymidine ratio observed in the nuclei early after infection. These findings may represent a true uncoating, resulting in the release of functional viral DNA, or a degradation of viral particles, because of their possible association with lysosomes (large-granule fraction) soon after infection.

It is reasonable to exclude the possibility that partially uncoated virus reaches the nucleus after being processed in the cytoplasm, because no changes in the buoyant density of the virions are detected in the nuclei until 4 hr postinfection. However, it cannot be ruled out that traces of naked viral DNA penetrate the nuclei, as may be suggested by the changes observed in the parental viral DNA at 2.5 hr after infection. At this time, the intranuclear uncoating has not yet started, but a small amount of ^{3}H-thymidine-labeled material sedimenting at the bottom of the gradient may represent free viral DNA. On the other hand, the difficulty in exactly reproducing the time sequence of the early events, probably due to the different batches of AGMK cells used, may explain the variations observed in different experiments when the intranuclear uncoating of the virus or the fate of the parental viral DNA was followed. These results suggest that the products of uncoating in the nuclei originate from the intranuclear viral particles, even though small amounts of viral proteins and DNA can be transferred separately from the cytoplasm to the nucleus. The last steps of uncoating of adenovirus type 5 are also performed in the nucleus (11).

Although small amounts of viral DNA (1% of the total intracellular radioactivity) are released from the cells into the medium, the cell surface does not seem to be involved in the uncoating phenomenon [in contrast to what has been reported for enteroviruses (4, 16; V. F. Chan and F. L. Black, Fed. Proc. **28**:433, 1969)], since the production of infectious SV40 was not decreased by treatment of the cells with deoxyribonuclease during the period of virus adsorption (*unpublished observations*).

Thus, it seems most likely that SV40 replication is initiated by the virus which reaches the nucleus.

After uncoating, the parental viral DNA seems to form a complex with cellular or newly synthesized viral proteins. With the sequence of changes of the parental SV40 DNA in the nuclei during and after uncoating, a gradual conversion of component I to component II of SV40 DNA occurs. This represents breaks in the circular structure of the viral genome (19), probably caused by a nickase in order to allow replication of the viral DNA.

An increase, up to 25 hr after infection, in the radioactive material recovered at the bottom of the gradient most likely indicates a progressive degradation of viral DNA with subsequent reutilization of the labeled precursor for cellular DNA synthesis. Further investigation could elucidate whether the 76S component appearing 2.5 hr after infection is of viral origin and whether it is related to the replicative form of SV40 DNA.

Finally, the possibility must be considered that the parental viral coat proteins present in the nuclei, where the viral genome expresses its genetic information, may play some role in the regulation of the transcription and replication of viral DNA.

ACKNOWLEDGMENTS

This investigation was supported by Public Health Service research grants PO1-CA 10815 and RO1-CA 04534 from the National Cancer Institute and SO1-FR-05549 from the General Research Support Branch, and by a research grant (E-89) from the American Cancer Society, Inc.

We thank Frantisek Sokol for helpful discussions. The excellent technical assistance of Johanna Snikkers, Marguarite Solomon, and Masatoshi Nagase is gratefully acknowledged.

LITERATURE CITED

1. Borun, T. W., M. D. Scharff, and E. Robbins. 1967. Preparation of mammalian polyribosomes with the detergent Nonidet P-40. Biochim. Biophys. Acta 149:302–304.
2. Crawford, L. V., and P. H. Black. 1964. The nucleic acid of simian virus 40. Virology 24:388–392.
3. Dales, S. 1965. Penetration of animal viruses into cells. Progr. Med. Virol. 7:1–43.
4. Holland, J. J. 1962. Irreversible eclipse of poliovirus by HeLa cells. Virology 16:163–176.
5. Holtzman, E., I. Smith, and S. Penman. 1966. Electron microscopic studies of detergent-treated HeLa cell nuclei. J. Mol. Biol. 17:131–135.
6. Hummeler, K., N. Tomassini, and F. Sokol. 1970. Morphological aspects of the uptake of simian virus 40 by permissive cells. J. Virol. 6:87–93.
7. Ifft, J. B., D. H. Voet, and J. Vinograd. 1961. The determination of density distributions of density gradients in binary solutions at equilibrium in the ultracentrifuge. J. Phys. Chem. 65:1138–1145.
8. Jensen, F., A. J. Girardi, R. V. Gilden, and H. Koprowski. 1964. Infection of human and simian tissue cultures with Rous sarcoma virus. Proc. Nat. Acad. Sci. U.S.A. 52:53–59.
9. Joklik, W. K. 1964. The intracellular uncoating of poxvirus DNA. I. The fate of radioactively-labeled rabbit poxvirus. J. Mol. Biol. 8:263–276.
10. Lawrence, W. C., and H. S. Ginsberg. 1967. Intracellular uncoating of type 5 adenovirus deoxyribonucleic acid. J. Virol. 1:851–867.

11. Lonberg-Holm, K., and L. Philipson. 1969. Early events of virus-cell interaction in an adenovirus system. J. Virol. 4:323–338.

12. Martin, R. G., and B. N. Ames. 1961. A method for determining the sedimentation behavior of enzymes: application to protein mixtures. J. Biol. Chem. 236:1372–1379.

13. O'Brien, B. R. A. 1964. The partial cytolysis of the amphibian erythrocytes and liver parenchyma cells by a nonionogenic surface active agent. J. Cell Biol. 20:521–524.

14. Ozer, H. L., and K. K. Takemoto. 1969. Site of host restriction of simian virus 40 mutants in an established African green monkey kidney cell line. J. Virol. 4:408–415.

15. Penman, S. 1969. p. 35–48. In K. Habel and N. P. Salzman (ed.), Fundamental techniques in virology. Academic Press Inc., New York.

16. Philipson, L., and M. Lind. 1964. Enterovirus eclipse in a cell free system. Virology 23:322–332.

17. Silverstein, S. C., and S. Dales. 1968. The penetration of reovirus RNA and initiation of its genetic functions in L-strain fibroblasts. J. Cell Biol. 36:197–230.

18. Swetly, P., G. Barbanti-Brodano, B. Knowles, and H. Koprowski. 1969. Response of simian virus 40-transformed cell lines and cell hybrids to superinfection with simian virus 40 and its deoxyribonucleic acid. J. Virol. 4:348–355.

19. Vinograd, J., J. Lebowitz, R. Radloff, R. Watson, and P. Laipis. 1965. The twisted circular form of polyoma viral DNA. Proc. Nat. Acad. Sci. U.S.A. 53:1104–1111.

Chromosomal Changes in Syrian Hamster Cells Transformed by Simian Virus 40 (SV40) and Variants of Defective SV40 (PARA)[1]

Maurice Nachtigal, Joseph L. Melnick, *and* Janet S. Butel

SOON AFTER the demonstration that simian virus 40 (SV40) could transform Syrian hamster cells *in vitro* (*1–3*), the resulting transformed cells were shown to contain many different types of structural chromosome aberrations and to develop heteroploid stemlines (*4*). In 1964, it was found that a particular strain of adenovirus type 7 carried defective SV40 genomes encased in adenovirus capsids (*5–7*). The particle containing the defective SV40 genetic information, called PARA (*8*), could transform Syrian hamster cells *in vitro* (*9*). Black and White (*10*) showed that Syrian hamster kidney cells transformed *in vitro* by

---

[1] Supported in part by Public Health Service research grant CA 04600 from the National Cancer Institute.

different transcapsidant populations of PARA-adenoviruses had chromosomal damage similar to that found in SV40-transformed cells but different from the stable karyotype of adenovirus 12-transformed cells.

Our study analyzes the chromosomal changes occurring in Syrian hamster kidney and lung cells inoculated with SV40 and different variants of PARA-adenoviruses. The isolates of PARA varied with respect to: 1) localization of the SV40 tumor (T) antigen induced during the lytic cycle (*11*, *12*) and in transformed cells (*13–15*), and 2) their tumor-inducing potential in newborn Syrian hamsters (*11*, *16*).

MATERIALS AND METHODS

Viruses.—Two different strains of SV40—the Baylor strain SV40 (By) (*17*, *18*) and SV40 (Bp), obtained from the Budapest Institute of Hygiene (*19*), were used after 8 passages in CV-1 cells and 5 passages in R-ICA cells, respectively. Five variants of PARA-adenovirus 7, derived from the parental LL strain of adenovirus type 7 (*5–7*) by 2 successive plaque purifications in green monkey kidney (GMK) cells (*11*), were used after 2–4 passages in GMK cells. The PARA-adenovirus 16 was obtained by transcapsidation (*8*), from the parental PARA-adenovirus (*16*). Table 1 summarizes the pertinent characteristics of the viruses.

Cell lines.—Of 15 cell lines studied for chromosomes, 14 transformed after exposure to SV40 or PARA-adenoviruses and 1 transformed spontaneously. Details concerning the transformation experiments and characteristics of the transformed cell lines (*15*, *20–22*) are given in table 2. Cell lines SHL-7 (73), SHL-7 (10), SHL-7 (39), SHL-7 (1cT), SHL-7 (2cT), and SHL-16 were established from adult Syrian hamster lung cells transformed by PARA-adenoviruses, line SHL-S (By) was from SV40-exposed adult Syrian hamster lung cells, and line SHL-S (Bp) was from newborn Syrian hamster lung cells that transformed after inoculation with SV40.

164

TABLE 1.—Properties of viruses used to obtain transformed Syrian hamster cell lines

Virus	Strain	Oncogenicity in Syrian hamsters	Transformation of Syrian hamster cells	Localization of SV40 T antigen in GMK cells	References
SV40	Baylor	++	++	Nucleus	(17, 18)
SV40	Budapest	++	++	Nucleus	(19)
PARA-adenovirus 7	Clone 73nT	0	+++	Nucleus	(11, 15, 20)
PARA-adenovirus 7	Clone 10nT	0	+++	Nucleus	(11, 15, 20)
PARA-adenovirus 7	Clone 39nT	0	+++	Nucleus	(11, 15, 20)
PARA-adenovirus 7	Clone 1cT	+0	++	Cytoplasm	(11–13, 15, 20)
PARA-adenovirus 7	Clone 2cT	0	++	Cytoplasm	(11–15, 20)
PARA-adenovirus 16			+	Nucleus	(15, 16, 20)

Cell lines SHK-7 (73), SHK-7 (10), SHK-7 (39), and SHK-7 (2cT) originated from adult Syrian hamster kidney cells transformed by different variants of PARA-adenovirus 7. Cell lines SHK-S (Bp) and SHE-S (Bp) were obtained by transformation with SV40 of adult Syrian hamster kidney cells and of Syrian hamster embryo cells, respectively. A Syrian hamster embryo cell line (SHE), which "transformed" spontaneously, and Syrian hamster lung cells (SHL), obtained from an adult animal, were included as controls. All cell lines were maintained in culture containing Eagle's medium, supplemented with 10% fetal calf serum, 0.075% bicarbonate, 100 U/ml penicillin, 100 μg/ml streptomycin, and 50 μg/ml each of fungizone and mycostatin.

Chromosome analysis.—Cells growing in 8-ounce prescription bottles were used to obtain chromosomes for analysis. Chromosomes were usually prepared 48 hours after subcultivation of the cells. For several passages before chromosome analysis, the anti-PPLO agent Tylocine (Grand Island Biological Co., Grand Island, N.Y.) was incorporated into the culture medium. Three hours before fixation, colchicine was added to the culture medium at a final concentration of 50 μg/ml, and the cultures were incubated for 2 hours at 37°C. The medium was removed and replaced with 4 ml of 0.05% trypsin–0.02% Versene solution. Incubation was continued at 37°C until the cells detached from the glass (approximately 20 minutes). At that time, 1 ml growth medium and 15 ml distilled water were added to the cell suspension, and the mixture was left standing at room temperature for 30 minutes. Thereafter, the cells were sedimented in a clinical centrifuge and the supernatant was poured off. The button of sedimented cells was then resuspended into the few drops of residual fluid by gentle agitation of the centrifuge tube.

Freshly prepared fixative (1 volume glacial acetic acid mixed with 3 volumes cooled absolute methanol) was added dropwise to the cell suspension to a final volume of approximately 3 ml, and the mixture was placed at 4°C for at least 30

166

TABLE 2.—Properties of Syrian hamster cell lines examined for chromosome constitution

Cell line	Transforming virus	Origin of cells	Unlimited growth of cells *in vitro*		Morphology	Piling-up	SV40 T antigen		Transplantability in Syrian hamsters
			Crisis	No crisis			Present	Localization	
SHL-7 (73)	PARA (73nT)-adeno 7	Adult lung	0	+	Fibroblastic	+	+	Nucleus	High
SHL-7 (10)	PARA (10nT)-adeno 7	Adult lung	+	0	Fibroblastic	+	+	Nucleus	Intermediate
SHL-7 (39)	PARA (39nT)-adeno 7	Adult lung	+	0	Fibroblastic	+	+	Nucleus	Very low
SHL-7 (1cT)	PARA (1cT)-adeno 7	Adult lung	+	0	Fibroblastic	+	+	Cytoplasm	Very low
SHL-7 (2cT)	PARA (2cT)-adeno 7	Adult lung	0	+	Fibroblastic	+	+	Nucleus	High
SHL-16	PARA-adeno 16	Adult lung	+	0	Fibroblastic	+	+	Nucleus	Very high
SHL-S (By)	SV40 (Baylor)	Newborn lung	+	0	Epithelial	0	0	—	None
SHL-S (Bp)	SV40 (Budapest)	Adult kidney	0	+	Fibroblastic	+	+	Nucleus	None
SHK-7 (73)	PARA (73nT)-adeno 7	Adult kidney	0	+	Fibroblastic	+	+	Nucleus	Very High
SHK-7 (10)	PARA (10nT)-adeno 7	Adult kidney	0	+	Fibroblastic	+	+	Nucleus	None
SHK-7 (39)	PARA (39nT)-adeno 7	Adult kidney	0	+	Fibroblastic	+	+	Nucleus	Intermediate
SHK-7 (2cT)	PARA (2cT)-adeno 7	Adult kidney	0	+	Epithelial	+	+	Cytoplasm	High
SHE-S (Bp)	SV40 (Budapest)	Total embryo	+	0	Epithelial	0	0	Nucleus	Very low
SHE-S (Bp)	SV40 (Budapest)	Total embryo	0	+	Fibroblastic	0	0	—	None
SHE	Not exposed		0	0		0	0	—	None
SHL	Not exposed	Adult lung	0	0	Fibroblastic	0	0	—	None

minutes. The cells were then resedimented, the fixative was changed as described, and the suspension was held overnight at 4°C. The next day, the fixative was changed at least 2 times. Five or six drops of cell suspension were then placed on wet, very clean microscope slides and the cell film was air-dried. The slides were stained with 10% Giemsa solution in distilled water for 10–15 minutes, washed under running tap water, dried, and mounted with Permount.

Metaphases were examined with the oil immersion objective. All metaphases were drawn by hand and the exact number of chromosomes was recorded. All structural chromosome abnormalities were also recorded, as were the number of identifiable X, D, E, and F chromosomes of the normal Syrian hamster karyotype (23, 24). Whenever necessary, karyotypes were prepared from magnified reprints of photographed metaphases. In evaluation of the incidence of chromosome abnormalities, 3 categories were considered: 1) breaks, including chromatid, chromosome, and isochromatidic breaks, and acentric and double fragments; 2) dicentrics, including tricentric or polycentric chromosomes and rejoinings; and 3) double minutes, typical minute double-chromatin bodies described by Cox et al. (25), Mark (26), and Levan et al. (27).

RESULTS

Chromosome Constitution of Syrian Hamster Cell Lines Which Transformed After Exposure to SV40

Four cell lines that transformed after inoculation with SV40 were examined for chromosomes (table 3). SHL-S (By) and SHL-S (Bp), of lung origin, showed no specific evidence of the viral genome because the "transformed" cells lacked the T antigen marker. The only evidence that these lines were virus transformed was their continued growth after exposure to SV40, while parallel, nonexposed lung cell cultures did not survive. They were included, however, to determine whether their chromosome constitutions shared any similarities

168

with those of transformed cell lines containing SV40-induced antigens.

The SHL-S (By) cells had a normal diploid chromosome complement. SHK-S (Bp) cells also tended to maintain near-diploid chromosome numbers for many passages after virus inoculation. However, in all passages of this cell line examined, there were considerable variation and spreading in the distribution of chromosome numbers. Cell lines SHL-S (Bp) and SHE-S (Bp) converted to hypotetraploid stemlines.

At passage 20, the number of D chromosomes increased in about 50% of the diploid and hyperdiploid SHK-S (Bp) cells and in hyperdiploid cells at passage 45, but no X chromosome was seen. The hypotetraploid SHE-S (Bp) cells showed 1 X, 14–16 D, 6 E, and 5–6 F chromosomes. A similar increase in the E and F chromosomes, found in hypertriploid-hypotetraploid SHK-S (Bp) cells, was associated with a significant decrease in the number of D chromosomes.

Structural Chromosome Aberrations in Syrian Hamster Cell Lines Which Transformed After Exposure to SV40

The level of cells with breaks was relatively low ($\leq$ 15%) in all the SV40-transformed cell lines, including the lines containing intranuclear SV40 T antigen and the 2 hamster lung cell lines which "transformed" after exposure to SV40 but lacking detectable amounts of T antigen (text-fig. 1).

The frequency of cells with dicentric chromosomes was between 10 and 20% in the SV40-transformed Syrian hamster kidney and embryo cell lines (text-fig. 2). Lung cell line SHL-S (Bp) showed a similar proportion of dicentric chromosomes soon after exposure to SV40. However, in later passages this line was like the other SV40-exposed "transformed" lung cell line, SHL-S (By), in that both contained between 0 and 8% cells with this particular chromosome aberration.

Certain passages of the SHK-S (Bp) and SHE-S (Bp) cell lines had a high percentage of double-

169

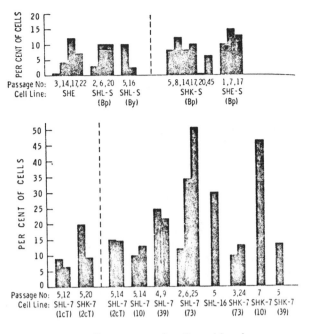

TEXT-FIGURE 1.—Frequency of cells with chromosome breaks in Syrian hamster cells transformed either spontaneously or after exposure to SV40 or PARA-adenovirus hybrid populations.

minute chromosomes (text-fig. 3). The appearance of this chromosome aberration was concomitant with the development of hypotetraploid cell stemlines. In the SHK-S (Bp) line, the double minutes reached a level of 30% of the cells examined at passage 45. At this passage, 50% of the cells were in the hypertriploid-hypotetraploid range and all the double minutes were in this group of cells.

Chromosome Constitution of Syrian Hamster Cell Lines Transformed by PARA-Adenovirus Populations

Passages of 10 PARA-transformed adult Syrian hamster cell lines, 6 of lung and 4 of kidney origin,

TABLE 3.—Distribution of chromosome numbers in Syrian hamster cell lines which "transformed" either spontaneously or after exposure to SV40

Cell line	Pas- sage No.	40	41	42	43	44	45	46	47	48	49	50	51– 55	56– 60	61– 65	66– 70	71– 75	76– 80	81– 85	86– 90	91– 95	96– 100	>100	Total No. of cells ana- lyzed
SHL-S (By)	5		1	1	5	*43*	1																	52
	16		1	1	9	*27*																		40
SHL-S (Bp)	2				2	4	3												3					15
	6		1											1				5	*15*	2				20
	20																		13	3	6	1	2	53
SHK-S (Bp)	5	3	2	3	2	6	1	5	2	3	3	1	1		2	4	9	5	2	1	6	1	2	50
	8	2	2	2	6	4	4	6	3	2		1	2	1	2	2	2	*21*	2	2	3	1	1	53
	14	1	3	8	11	9	3						1	3	2	1		2	3	2	3		3	53
	17		2	3	8	1	9	3	2	1						4	1	1	7	4	2			50
	20		2	4	9	8	5	13						1	1	4	5	2	7	4		2		60
	45	1				*37*	2	4	2								1	*19*	1	1		1	1	51
SHE-S (Bp)	1	2			4					1				1	1	3	1	1	1	2	1			30
	7																2	7	*13*	5	2	2	2	47
	17																3	4	8	4	2	2	4	35
SHE	3		2	6	7	*21*	1	1												1				23
	14		1	1	1	*18*	3												3	5				31
	17	2		6	10	*25*	1								1				1	4				25
	22			1	6	*12*	2												5	5				50
SHL	6	2	2	2	5	*15*													2	3	1			30
																								22

171

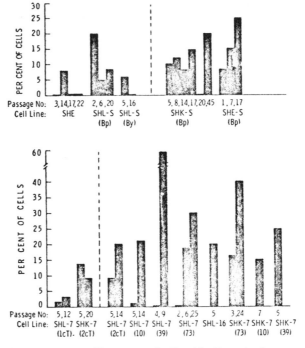

TEXT-FIGURE 2.—Frequency of cells with dicentric chromosomes in Syrian hamster cells transformed either spontaneously or after exposure to SV40 or PARA-adenovirus hybrid populations.

were examined for chromosomes. A significant proportion of cells with the normal chromosome number was found in different passages of the SHL-7 (73) and SHL-7 (10) lines, as well as in early passages of the SHL-7 (39), SHL-7 (2cT), and SHK-7 (2cT) lines (table 4). Lines SHL-7 (1cT) and SHK-7 (10) were hypodiploid and lines SHL-7 (39) and SHL-7 (2cT) tended to develop hypodiploid stemlines. Four cell lines had modal numbers in the hypotetraploid range: SHL-16 and SHK-7 (39) at early passages and SHK-7 (73) and SHK-7 (2cT) at later passages.

At passages 2 and 6, a predominantly normal number of X, D, E, and F chromosomes were in SHL-7 (73) cells having a diploid chromosome

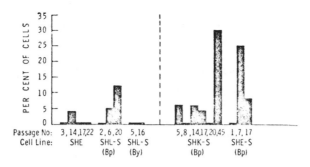

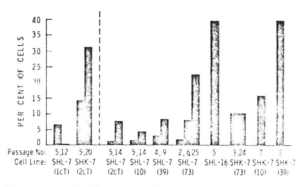

TEXT-FIGURE 3.—Frequency of cells with double-minute chromosomes in Syrian hamster cells transformed either spontaneously or after exposure to SV40 or PARA-adenovirus hybrid populations.

complement, but at passage 25, all cells having 44 chromosomes lacked at least 1 D chromosome and had extra F chromosomes. At least 50% of the diploid SHL-7 (10) cells had the normal number of identifiable chromosomes, and no marker chromosome was evident. D chromosomes decreased in approximately 80% of diploid SHL-7 (39) cells at passage 4. Almost all hypodiploid cells of these 2 cell lines lacked at least 1 D chromosome. At passage 5, modal SHL-7 (lcT) cells with 40 chromosomes consistently had only 6 D chromosomes, missing 2; at passage 12, 30% of the cells had only 5 D chromosomes. At passage 14, SHL-7

173

(2cT) cells tended to miss 1 D chromosome, and at passage 7, 75% of the SHK-7 (10) hypodiploid cells and 50% of the diploid cells also had fewer D chromosomes. The hypotetraploid SHK-7 (73) cells at passage 24 had only 3 F chromosomes. One F chromosome was lost in all diploid SHK-7 (2cT) cells at passage 5, and at passage 20 most hypotetraploid cells had only 2 F chromosomes. One F chromosome was also missing in more than 50% of the SHL-7 (39) cells at passage 9.

Structural Chromosome Aberrations in Syrian Hamster Cell Lines Transformed by PARA-Adenovirus Populations

Cells containing chromosome breaks were often found in the SHK-7 (2cT), SHL-7 (39), SHL-7 (73), SHL-16, and SHK-7 (10) lines in early passages after transformation (text-fig. 1). The values obtained with these lines, which had not undergone more than 7 passages *in vitro*, ranged from 20–45%. The lowest level of chromosome breaks ($\leq 8\%$) was consistently found in the SHL-7 (1cT) line (text-fig. 1).

Early passages of the SHL-7 (1cT), SHL-7 (10), and SHL-7 (39) cell lines showed almost no dicentric chromosomes ($\leq 2\%$) (text-fig. 2). The highest levels of cells containing dicentric chromosomes (15–25%) soon after transformation (5–7 passages) were observed in the SHK-7 (39), SHK-7 (10), SHL-16, and SHL-7 (73) lines (text-fig. 2). Lines SHL-7 (10), SHL-7 (39), and SHK-7 (73) showed a striking increase in the frequency of dicentric chromosomes after further subcultivation *in vitro* (text-fig. 2). At passage 9 of the SHL-7 (39) cells, 60% contained this aberration. In both kidney and lung cells transformed by variants of PARA and containing intranuclear SV40 T antigen, cells containing dicentrics increased. In contrast, 2 PARA-transformed cell lines with SV40 T antigen in the cytoplasm, SHL-7 (1cT) of lung origin and SHK-7 (2cT) of kidney origin, showed somewhat lower levels of dicentrics.

174

TABLE 4.—Distribution of chromosome numbers in Syrian hamster cell lines transformed by PARA-adenovirus hybrid populations

Cell line	Passage No.							Chromosome numbers																Total No. of cells analyzed
		38	39	40	41	42	43	44	45	46	47	48	51–55	56–60	61–65	66–70	71–75	76–80	81–85	86–90	91–96	96–100	>100	
SHL-7(73)	2					3	10	29	2	5													1	50
	6				2	2	4	17	7	6	2							2	2	4		1	1	50
	25				3	3	4	7	3	6	1	1					1			2				31
SHL-7(10)	5					4	5	24	13	1	4													51
	14			2		1	6	8	2	2								2						23
SHL-7(39)	4	1			2	1	7	16	9	1														37
	9				15	8	11	10	1	2	4													51
SHL-7(1cT)	5		11	21	6	3	1											3					1	46
	12		6	15	4	2	2											1						30
SHL-7(2cT)	5				1	2	7	20	17	3									3					53
	14					15	2	11	4	3	3			2	3	2		7		2				54
SHL-16	5							6	5	8	4		2	2	1	2		5		1				36
SHK-7(73)	3																1	7	22					30
	24																5	5	20					30
SHK-7(10)	7				6	12	25	7		1					1									52
	5												2	2	3	4	4	6	28	4	1			54
SHK-7(39)	5				2	4	4	13	2	3	3			2	1									34
SHK-7(2cT)	20												2	2	1	4	12	8	3					32

Cells with double-minute chromosomes were most frequent (about 38%) in the SHL-16 and SHK-7 (39) lines, both of which had hypotetraploid modal values (text-fig. 3). The incidence of this type of chromosome aberration increased in later passages of the SHL-7 (73) and SHK-7 (2cT) lines. In the latter line, this increase was associated with a shift toward a hypotetraploid stemline. However, in the SHL-7 (73) cells, >50% of the cells containing double minutes were hypodiploid.

Chromosome Constitution of a Syrian Hamster Embryo Cell Line Which Transformed Spontaneously

Chromosomes of the SHE line were analyzed at passages 3, 14, 17, and 22, which represented 10, 33, 43, and 53 weeks of life *in vitro*, respectively. At all passages, cells with the diploid chromosome number constituted the modal group, although a certain proportion of near-diploid or near-tetraploid cells was always present (table 3). At passage 3, 2 types of diploid cells were found—one with the normal number of identifiable chromosomes and another with a missing D chromosome. The ratio of these 2 cell types was about 3:2. At subsequent passages, cells with the normal karyotype became extremely rare; almost all modal cells were pseudodiploid, containing 44 chromosomes but missing 1 D chromosome.

Structural Chromosome Aberrations in a Syrian Hamster Embryo Cell Line Which Transformed Spontaneously

The SHE line of embryo cells was analyzed at intervals during a year of propagation *in vitro*. It consistently exhibited an extremely low level of any type of structural chromosome aberration (text-figs. 1–3).

DISCUSSION

The results obtained show that Syrian hamster lung and kidney cells which transformed after inoculation with SV40 or variants of PARA-adenovirus hybrid populations differed in their chromosome constitution, modal chromosome number, and frequency of different types of chromosomal aberrations. In general, there were more chromosome abnormalities in the cells transformed by variants of PARA (defective SV40) than in those transformed by complete SV40.

Early passages of lung cell lines transformed by 3 nononcogenic variants of PARA-adenovirus 7 (1cT, 10nT, and 39nT) had diploid or hypodiploid stemlines coupled with a very low incidence of dicentric and double-minute chromosomes. In contrast, 2 lung cell lines transformed by oncogenic variants of PARA-adenovirus 7 (2cT and 73nT), except for passage 2 of the SHL-7 (73) line, contained a higher frequency of dicentrics. However, it cannot be suggested that the nononcogenic variants exert lesser effects on the chromosomes of the cells they transform, because in later passages both the SHL-7 (10) and SHL-7 (39) cells showed an increase in the frequency of dicentric chromosomes, reaching the highest level in the SHL-7 (39) line. In addition, the SHL-7 (1cT) and SHL-7 (39) lines had modal chromosome values well below the diploid number. This suggests that considerable chromosome loss or restructuring had actually occurred.

Since early passages (≤ 5) of the SHL-7 (10), SHL-7 (39), and SHL-7 (1cT) cell lines were positive for SV40 T antigen, but practically free from structural chromosome aberrations, there probably is no immediate temporal relationship between the appearance of SV40 T antigen and that of dicentric chromosomes. In other cell lines positive for T antigen [e.g., SHL-16, SHK-7 (73), and SHK-7 (39)], many dicentric chromosomes were in early passages. Therefore, not all cells transformed by variants of PARA showed this lack of relationship. The oncogenicity of the transforming virus did not influence the time of appearance of dicentric chromosomes.

Among the PARA-transformed lung cell lines, the first to develop high transplantability was SHL-16. This line was composed of cells in the hypotetraploid range containing a high incidence of structural chromosome aberrations. The function, if any, of the helper adenovirus type 16 in the initiation of this cell line is unknown.

In PARA-transformed Syrian hamster kidney cells [except in the SHK-7 (2cT) cell line], the frequency of dicentric chromosomes was high, irrespective of the oncogenic potential *in vivo* of the transforming virus, and was similar to, or slightly higher than, the level of dicentrics found in Syrian hamster kidney and embryo cells transformed by SV40. A similar incidence of dicentrics in early passages of hamster kidney cells transformed by SV40 (*4*) and PARA was reported (*10*). It appears, therefore, that adult Syrian hamster lung cells are more liable than hamster kidney or embryo cells to exhibit different chromosomal changes after transformation by PARA.

The apparent involvement of the acrocentric D group chromosomes in numerical abnormalities is noteworthy. The cell lines transformed by variants of PARA tended to have fewer of these chromosomes. This observation correlates well with that of van Steenis (*28*) and Levan (*29*) who reported that most human tumors analyzed contained fewer acrocentric chromosomes of groups D and G.

That lines SHL-7 (1cT) and SHK-7 (2cT), which contained SV40 T antigen in the cytoplasm, did not show as pronounced an increase in the frequency of cells with dicentrics or breaks as most of the other PARA-transformed lines is interesting. They followed, instead, a pattern of chromosomal evolution more closely resembling that in the spontaneously "transformed" SHE Syrian hamster embryo cell line and in SHL-S (Bp) and SHL-S (By) SV40-exposed "transformed" Syrian hamster lung cell lines which failed to synthesize detectable levels of SV40 T antigen.

These findings suggest that the presence of SV40 T antigen in the nucleus of transformed cells may be associated with the formation of dicentric chromosomes, even though a direct temporal relationship was not apparent. Many more cell lines would have to be characterized to definitely establish such an association. It would be of interest to study human cells transformed by the cytoplasmic variants of PARA to determine if SV40 T antigen in the cytoplasm of such cells would still be associated with a decreased incidence of chromosomal aberrations. Such aberrations tend to be quite common after SV40 transformation of human cells (*30–32*).

The SHL-S (Bp) and SHL-S (By) cell lines more closely resembled the spontaneously "transformed" hamster embryo line, SHE, with respect to the frequency of dicentric chromosomes than the SV40-transformed cell lines synthesizing T antigen. Therefore, the role of SV40 in the origin of the lung cell lines remains obscure. We are left with the still unexplained fact that exposure of Syrian hamster lung cells to SV40 has repeatedly resulted in the establishment of cell lines devoid of SV40 T antigen with extended lifetimes *in vitro*, while control unexposed cells fail to survive (*15*).

REFERENCES

(*1*) Rabson AS, Kirschstein RL: Induction of malignancy *in vitro* in newborn hamster kidney tissue infected with simian vacuolating virus (SV40). Proc Soc Exp Biol Med 111:323–328, 1962

(*2*) Black PH, Rowe WP: Transformation in hamster kidney monolayers by vacuolating virus, SV–40. Virology 19:107–109, 1963

(*3*) Ashkenazi A, Melnick JL: Tumorigenicity of simian papovavirus SV40 and of virus-transformed cells. J Nat Cancer Inst 30:1227–1265, 1963

(4) COOPER HL, BLACK PH: Cytogenetic studies of hamster kidney cell cultures transformed by the simian vacuolating virus (SV40). J Nat Cancer Inst 30:1015–1043, 1963

(5) HUEBNER RJ, CHANOCK RM, RUBIN BA, et al: Induction by adenovirus type 7 of tumors in hamsters having the antigenic characteristics of SV40 virus. Proc Nat Acad Sci USA 52:1333–1340, 1964

(6) ROWE WP, BAUM SG: Evidence for a possible genetic hybrid between adenovirus type 7 and SV40 viruses. Proc Nat Acad Sci USA 52:1340–1347, 1964

(7) RAPP F, MELNICK JL, BUTEL JS, et al: The incorporation of SV40 genetic material into adenovirus 7 as measured by intranuclear synthesis of SV40 tumor antigen. Proc Nat Acad Sci USA 52:1348–1352, 1964

(8) RAPP F, BUTEL JS, MELNICK JL: SV40-adenovirus "hybrid" populations: Transfer of SV40 determinants from one type of adenovirus to another. Proc Nat Acad Sci USA 54:717–724, 1965

(9) BLACK PH, TODARO GJ: In vitro transformation of hamster and human cells with the adeno 7-SV 40 hybrid virus. Proc Nat Acad Sci USA 54:374–381, 1965

(10) BLACK PH, WHITE BJ: In vitro transformation by the adenovirus-SV40 hybrid viruses. II. Characteristics of the transformation of hamster cells by the adeno 2-, adeno 3-, and adeno 12-SV40 viruses. J Exp Med 125:629–646, 1967

(11) RAPP F, PAULUZZI S, BUTEL JS: Variation in properties of plaque progeny of PARA (defective simian papovavirus 40)-adenovirus 7. J Virol 4:626–631, 1969

(12) BUTEL JS, GUENTZEL MJ, RAPP F: Variants of defective simian papovavirus 40 (PARA) characterized by cytoplasmic localization of simian papovavirus 40 tumor antigen. J Virol 4:632–641, 1969

(13) DUFF R, RAPP F, BUTEL JS: Transformation of hamster cells by variants of PARA-adenovirus 7 able to induce SV40 tumor antigen in the cytoplasm. Virology 42:273–275, 1970

(14) RICHARDSON LS, BUTEL JS: Properties of transformed hamster cells containing SV40 tumor antigen in the cytoplasm. Int J Cancer 7:75–85, 1971

(15) NACHTIGAL M, BUTEL JS: Variation in response of Syrian hamster lung cells to complete or defective SV40 (PARA). Proc Soc Exp Biol Med 135:727–731, 1970

(16) RAPP F, JERKOFSKY M, MELNICK JL, et al: Variation in the oncogenic potential of human adenoviruses

carrying a defective SV40 genome (PARA).
J Exp Med 127:77–90, 1968

(*17*) RAPP F, KITAHARA T, BUTEL JS, et al: Synthesis of
SV40 tumor antigen during replication of simian
papovavirus (SV40). Proc Nat Acad Sci USA
52:1138–1142, 1964

(*18*) RAPP F, BUTEL JS, FELDMAN LA, et al: Differential
effects of inhibitors on the steps leading to the formation of SV40 tumor and virus antigens. J Exp Med
121:935–944, 1965

(*19*) NACHTIGAL M, SAHNAZAROV N, GRAFFE LH, et al:
Chromosomal changes during transformation of
fetal bovine kidney cells infected with SV40 virus.
Rev Roum Inframicrobiol 7:27–40, 1970

(*20*) BUTEL JS, TEVETHIA SS, NACHTIGAL M: Malignant
transformation *in vitro* by "non-oncogenic" variants
of defective SV40 (PARA). J Immun 106:969–974,
1971

(*21*) NACHTIGAL M, SAHNAZAROV N, GRAFFE LH, et al:
Spontaneous and SV40 virus-induced transforma-
tion of a golden hamster embryo cell line. Rev Roum
Inframicrobiol 7:15–26, 1970

(*22*) SAHNAZAROV N, NACHTIGAL M, GRAFFE LH, et al:
Sequence of alterations in the course of transformation induced by SV40 virus in adult golden hamster
kidney cell cultures. Rev Roum Inframicrobiol
7:87–99, 1970

(*23*) ISHIHARA T, MOORE GE, SANDBERG AA: Chromosome constitution of two tumors of the golden hamster. J Nat Cancer Inst 29:161–195, 1962

(*24*) LEHMAN JM, MACPHERSON I, MOORHEAD PS: Karyotype of the Syrian hamster. J Nat Cancer Inst 31:
639–650, 1963

(*25*) COX D, YUNCKEN C, SPRIGGS AI: Minute chromatin
bodies in malignant tumours of childhood. Lancet
2:55–58, 1965

(*26*) MARK J: Double-minutes—a chromosomal aberration in Rous sarcomas in mice. Hereditas (Lund)
57:1–22, 1967

(*27*) LEVAN A, MANOLOV G, CLIFFORD P: Chromosomes
of a human neuroblastoma: A new case with acces-
sory minute chromosomes. J Nat Cancer Inst
41:1377–1387, 1968

(*28*) VAN STEENIS H: Chromosomes and cancer. Nature
(London) 209:819–821, 1966

(*29*) LEVAN A: Non-random representation of chromosome
types in human tumor stemlines. Hereditas (Lund)
55:28–38, 1966

(*30*) YERGANIAN G, SHEIN HM, ENDERS JF: Chromosomal
disturbances observed in human fetal renal cells

transformed *in vitro* by simian virus 40 and carried in culture. Cytogenetics (Basel) 1:314–324, 1962

(*31*) MOORHEAD PS, SAKSELA E: Non-random chromosomal aberrations in SV40-transformed human cells. J Cell Comp Physiol 62:57–83, 1963

(*32*) GIRARDI AJ, WEINSTEIN D, MOORHEAD PS: SV40 transformation of human diploid cells. A parallel study of viral and karyological parameters. Ann Med Exp Fenn 44:242–254, 1966

AUTHOR INDEX

KEY-WORD TITLE INDEX